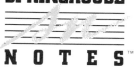

# SPRINGHOUSE

# N O T E S™

# NUTRITION AND DIET THERAPY

**Susan M. Quillman, RN, MN**
Ms. Quillman, the author of this book, is an Assistant Professor of Nursing at Northeast Louisiana University, Monroe, Louisiana. She earned her BSN from Northwestern State College, Natchitoches, Louisiana, and her MN from the University of Mississippi. Ms. Quillman is a member of the American Heart Association and the American Diabetes Association.

**Nancy R. Mitchell, RN, MSN**
Ms. Mitchell, the reviewer of this book, is an Assistant Professor at California State University at Bakersfield. She received her Diploma in nursing from Lincoln General School of Nursing at Lincoln, Nebraska. Later she earned her BSN from the University of Nebraska, Lincoln, and her MSN from the University of Texas, Austin. She is also a practicing medical-surgical nurse. Ms. Mitchell is a member of Sigma Theta Tau, the National Association of Orthopaedic Nurses, and the National League for Nursing.

Springhouse Corporation
Springhouse, Pennsylvania

# Staff

**Executive Director, Editorial**
Stanley Loeb

**Executive Director, Creative Services**
Jean Robinson

**Director of Trade and Textbooks**
Minnie B. Rose, RN, BSN, MEd

**Art Director**
John Hubbard

**Consultant**
Maryann Foley, RN, BSN

**Acquisitions Editor**
Donna L. Hilton, RN, BSN, CEN

**Editor**
Kevin Law

**Copy Editors**
David Prout (manager), Elizabeth Kiselev

**Designers**
Stephanie Peters (associate art director),
Julie Carleton Barlow

**Art Production**
Robert Perry (manager), Anna Brindisi, Donald
Knauss, Catherine Mace, Robert Wieder

**Typography**
David Kosten (manager), Diane Paluba (assistant
manager), Joyce Rossi Biletz, Brenda C. Mayer,
Robin Rantz, Brent Rinedoller, Valerie L. Rosenberger

**Manufacturing**
Deborah Meiris (manager), T.A. Landis, Jennifer Suter

**Production Coordination**
Aline S. Miller (manager), Maura C. Murphy

SN10-010789

Library of Congress Cataloging-in-Publication Data
Quillman, Susan M.
    Nutrition and diet therapy.
    (Springhouse notes)
    Bibliography: p.     Includes index.
    1. Nutrition—Outlines, syllabi, etc.    2. Diet therapy—Outlines, syllabi, etc.    3. Nursing—Outlines, syllabi, etc.    I. Title.    II. Series.
    RM216.Q55 1990        613.2        89-6027
    ISBN 0-87434-205-8

# Contents

# How to Use Springhouse Notes

Today, more than ever, nursing students face enormous time pressures. Nursing education has become more sophisticated, increasing the difficulties students have with studying efficiently and keeping pace.

The need for a comprehensive, well-deisgned series of study aids is great, which is why we've produced Springhouse Notes...to meet that need. Springhouse Notes provide essential course material in outline form, enabling the nursing student to study more effectively, improve understanding, achieve higher test scores, and get better grades.

Key features appear throughout each book, making the information more accessible and easier to remember.
• **Learning Objectives.** These objectives precede each section in the book to help the student evaluate knowledge before and after study.
• **Key Points.** Highlighted in color throughout the bok, these points provide a way to quickly review critical information. Key points may include:
—a cardinal sign or symptoms of a disorder
—the most current or popular theory about a topic
—a distinguishing characteristic of a disorder
—the most important step of a process
—a critical assessment component
—a crucial nursing intervention
—the most widely used or successful therapy or treatment
• **Points to Remember.** This information, found at the end of each section, summarizes the section in capsule form.
• **Glossary.** Difficult, frequently used, or sometimes misunderstood terms are defined for the student at the end of each section.

**Remember:** Springhouse Notes are learning tools designed to *help* you. They are not intended for use as a primary information source. They should never substitute for class attendance, text reading, or classroom note taking.

*Nutrition and Diet Therapy* uses the basic concepts of nutrition, energy, and metabolism, along with information on digestion and assimilation of essential nutrients and nutritional needs throughout the life cycle, as a framework for presenting diet therapy. Important areas such as anthropometry in nutritional assessment, specialized diets, malnutrition, and enteral and parenteral nutrition are discussed. Nutritional therapy sections use a nursing process approach and are organized around each affected nutrient. Information on each diet covers specific indications, foods to avoid and include, and nursing implications, which must always be adapted to meet the individual client's needs.

# Overview of Nutrition

**Learning Objectives**

After studying this section, the reader should be able to:

● Describe the relationship between nutrition and nutritional status.

● Identify the essential nutrients necessary for adequate nutrition.

● Describe the relationship between metabolism and energy.

● Discuss the factors that affect basal metabolic rate.

● Describe the factors that contribute to energy requirements.

## I. Overview of Nutrition

### A. Basic concepts

1. Nutrition is a combination of processes by which the body receives and uses nutrients
   a. Encompasses principles from the physical, biological, and behavioral sciences and the arts
   b. Concerned with those properties of food that build sound bodies and promote health
2. Nutritional status refers to the body condition that results from the use of available nutrients
3. Hunger is the physiologic response to the desire to consume food
   a. Associated with objective sensations, such as stomach contractions
   b. Integrated in the hypothalamus of the brain
4. Appetite is the desire to eat, which normally accompanies hunger
   a. Involves a pleasurable sensation
   b. Is influenced greatly by the person's perception of food
5. Satiety refers to the feeling of fullness or satisfaction that normally prompts a person to stop eating
6. Essential nutrients are those components of food necessary for growth and functioning that must be supplied in adequate amounts from ingestion of food. They include:
   a. Water
   b. Lipids
   c. Carbohydrates
   d. Proteins
   e. Vitamins
   f. Minerals
7. The functions of nutrients include:
   a. Providing energy
   b. Maintaining body tissues
   c. Acting in body processes, such as growth, cell activity, enzyme production, and temperature regulation

### B. Metabolism

1. General information
   a. Metabolism refers to the sum of all the chemical reactions that occur in the body's cells
   b. Hormones regulate metabolism
   c. Metabolism involves the action of specific enzymes to carry out specific processes
2. Phases
   a. *Anabolism* involves synthesis of cellular substances from nutrients and results in production of new, more complex substances and stored energy. This process is necessary for tissue growth, maintenance, and repair

   b. *Catabolism* involves the breakdown of cellular substances to release energy
3. Factors affecting metabolism
   a. Amount of food consumed. Excessive food consumption results in an increase in adipose tissue development, leading to increased anabolism; limited food intake leads to catabolism
   b. Activity level. Rest increases anabolism; exercise increases catabolism
   c. Physical stress. Fever, burns, fractures, and exposure to toxins increase catabolism
   d. Hormones such as growth hormone, male sex hormone, and thyroid hormone increase catabolism

## C. Energy
1. General information
   a. Energy production occurs as a by-product of carbohydrate, lipid, and protein metabolism in the form of adenosine triphosphate (ATP)
   b. Energy is measured in kilocalories, commonly referred to as calories
2. Energy value of nutrients
   a. Carbohydrates yield approximately 4 calories per gram
   b. Lipids yield approximately 9 calories per gram
   c. Proteins yield approximately 4 calories per gram
3. Total energy requirements
   a. The body normally uses carbohydrates as its primary source of energy, followed by lipids and then proteins
   b. The body draws on its stored energy reserves, such as glycogen stored in the liver, fat stored in adipose tissue, and protein stored as fatty acids, if dietary intake doesn't meet energy needs
   c. Factors influencing total energy requirements include basal metabolic rate, physical activity, and the specific dynamic action (SDA) of ingested foods
4. Energy balance
   a. Energy balance occurs when the caloric intake from food equals the caloric requirements that maintain body processes and fuel physical activity
   b. Weight gain occurs when caloric intake exceeds requirements; then excess calories are stored as fat
   c. Weight loss occurs when caloric intake is less than caloric requirements

## D. Basal metabolic rate (BMR)
1. General information
   a. BMR is the minimum energy required to maintain essential life processes when the body is at rest
   b. BMR is determined by the amount of oxygen used by body tissues, and is expressed as calories consumed per hour per square meter of body surface area or per kilogram of body weight

    2.  Factors affecting BMR

        a.  Age. BMR is highest during periods of rapid growth, chiefly in the first and second years of life and in the prepubertal years

        b.  Body composition. BMR decreases with increased adipose tissue

        c.  Body surface area. BMR increases with increased body surface area

        d.  Sex. In persons of equal height and weight, women have a 5% to 10% lower BMR than men

        e.  Sleep. During sleep, BMR is 10% to 15% below normal waking levels

        f.  Climate. Persons living in warmer climates generally have a 10% lower BMR than those in colder climates

**E. Application to nursing**

    1.  General information

        a.  The desire for food is a basic human need

        b.  Good nutrition is essential in promoting health, preventing illness, and restoring health after illness or injury

        c.  Inadequate nutrition makes optimal health impossible

    2.  Nursing implications

        a.  Use a knowledge of nutrition to promote health through education and counseling of both well and ill clients

        b.  Apply the scientific principles of nutrition to promote health and prevent illness

        c.  Help feed clients who need assistance

        d.  Influence clients' food choices in a nutritionally sound manner

        e.  Encourage clients to consume appropriate types and amounts of food

        f.  Motivate clients to modify diet to promote health

## Points to Remember

Nutrition is a combination of processes by which the body receives and uses nutrients; the study of nutrition is concerned with those properties of food that build sound bodies and promote health.

Nutritional status refers to the body condition that results from the use of available nutrients.

Essential nutrients are components of ingested food that are necessary for growth and functioning when supplied in adequate amounts. They include water, lipids, carbohydrates, proteins, vitamins, and minerals.

Energy is produced by the metabolism of carbohydrates, lipids, and proteins.

## Glossary

**Enzyme**—substance that initiates and accelerates a chemical reaction

**Hormone**—chemical substance produced by an endocrine gland that has a specific regulatory effect on other body cells

**Nutrient**—component of food that provides nourishment and affects the body's nutritive or metabolic processes

**Specific dynamic action (SDA)**—increased heat production resulting from the metabolism of food

# Digestive System

**Learning Objectives**

After studying this section, the reader should be able to:

- Describe the parts of the digestive system.

- Identify the functions of the digestive system.

- Describe the parts of the alimentary canal.

- Identify the functions of the various parts of the alimentary canal.

- Describe the accessory organs.

- Identify the functions of the accessory organs as they relate to digestion.

## II. Digestive System

### A. Introduction

1. The digestive system is composed of the alimentary canal and accessory organs
2. The alimentary canal is the tubular structure that begins at the mouth and ends at the anal canal and includes the mouth, pharynx, esophagus, stomach, and small and large intestines
3. The accessory organs aid in the digestive process and include the salivary glands, liver, gallbladder, and pancreas
4. Functions of the digestive system include:
   a. Ingestion of food
   b. Transportation of food substances and waste products
   c. Secretion of acid, mucus, digestive enzymes, and bile
   d. Digestion of food particles into soluble materials
   e. Absorption of soluble materials
   f. Storage of waste products from digestion
   g. Elimination of waste products from the body

### B. Mouth (buccal cavity)

1. General information
   a. Formed by the cheeks, hard and soft palates, tongue, and teeth
   b. Contains the taste buds, located in the tongue, and the salivary glands
2. Functions
   a. Receives food to be ingested
   b. Masticates food through the action of the teeth and jaw
   c. Receives salivary amylase (ptyalin) from the salivary glands
   d. Mixes food with saliva, mucus, and digestive enzymes
   e. Initiates the swallowing process of food particles from the mouth

### C. Pharynx

1. General information
   a. Is a tubelike structure
   b. Extends from the back of the mouth (at the level of the base of the skull) to the esophagus
2. Function: Serves as a passageway for both respiratory and digestive tracts

### D. Esophagus

1. General information
   a. Is a collapsible tube that lies posterior to the trachea and heart
   b. Extends from the pharynx to the stomach
2. Functions
   a. Acts as a passageway for food from the pharynx to the stomach
   b. Contracts during swallowing and moves the food mass with the aid of secretions from the mucous glands

c.  Allows entrance of the food mass into the stomach when the gastroesophageal sphincter relaxes

## E.  Stomach
1.  General information
    a.  Is an elongated, pouchlike structure that lies in the upper part of the abdominal cavity under the liver and diaphragm
    b.  Is divided into three sections: fundus, body, and antrum
    c.  Contains the cardiac and pyloric sphincters
2.  Functions
    a.  Serves as a reservoir, storing the food mass until it is partially digested
    b.  Secretes gastric juices
    c.  Breaks the food mass into smaller particles and mixes them with gastric juices to form chyme
    d.  Carries on a limited amount of absorption of certain substances, such as alcohol and aspirin
    e.  Controls the emptying of chyme from the stomach to the small intestine, through the pyloric sphincter

## F.  Small intestine
1.  General information
    a.  Is a tubelike structure approximately 20′ (6 m) in length; fills most of the abdominal cavity
    b.  Is divided into three sections: duodenum, jejunum, and ileum
2.  Functions
    a.  Secretes hormones, mucus, and enzymes
    b.  Completes a major part of the digestive process
    c.  Absorbs most of the end products of digestion into the blood and lymph

## G.  Liver
1.  General information
    a.  Is part of the biliary system
    b.  Is the largest gland in the body, weighing between 3 and 4 lb (1.4 and 1.8 kg)
    c.  Is located mainly on the right side of the abdominal cavity, below the diaphragm
    d.  Consists of liver lobules (the basic functioning unit of the liver) and a system of ducts
2.  Functions
    a.  Assists in metabolizing proteins, fats, and carbohydrates
    b.  Synthesizes proteins
    c.  Stores such substances as iron and vitamins A, $B_{12}$, and D
    d.  Detoxifies toxins and drugs
    e.  Produces bile

**H. Gallbladder**
   1.  General information
      a.  Is part of the biliary system
      b.  Consists of a pear-shaped sac located on the undersurface of the liver
   2.  Functions
      a.  Concentrates and stores bile from the liver
      b.  Contracts and ejects concentrated bile for delivery into the duodenum when needed for digestion

**I.  Pancreas**
   1.  General information
      a.  Is part of the biliary system
      b.  Is shaped roughly like a fish; located posterior to the stomach
      c.  Contains both endocrine and exocrine tissues
   2.  Functions
      a.  Secretes pancreatic juice from the exocrine cells
      b.  Secretes insulin from beta endocrine cells
      c.  Secretes glucagon from alpha endocrine cells

**J.  Large intestine**
   1.  General information
      a.  Is a large tube averaging approximately 2½″ (6.4 cm) in diameter and approximately 5′ to 6′ (1.5 to 1.8 m) in length
      b.  Extends from the ileocecal valve to the anus
      c.  Is divided into cecum; ascending, transverse, descending, and sigmoid colons; rectum; and anus
   2.  Functions
      a.  Absorbs water and some electrolytes
      b.  Stores waste products from digestion temporarily until evacuation occurs
      c.  Eliminates waste products from the body via the anus

## Points to Remember

The digestive system is composed of the alimentary canal and four accessory organs.

The alimentary canal includes the mouth, pharynx, esophagus, stomach, small intestine (duodenum, jejunum, ileum), and large intestine (cecum, colon, rectum, anus).

The accessory organs include the salivary glands and the biliary system.

The biliary system is composed of the liver, gallbladder, and pancreas.

Digestion begins in the mouth with the ingestion of food, the chewing of food, and the action of saliva.

If the digestive system is not functioning properly, the body may be unable to receive or use adequate amounts of nutrients to meet its requirements.

## Glossary

**Bile**—fluid produced by the liver that is concentrated and stored in the gallbladder

**Chyme**—semifluid paste of food particles and gastric juices

**Mastication**—process of chewing, grinding, or tearing food with teeth while mixing the food with saliva

**Sphincter**—circular muscle at the entrance and exit of the stomach that allows substances to pass through but prevents backflow

# Digestion of Nutrients

## Learning Objectives

After studying this section, the reader should be able to:

• Define digestion.

• Describe the digestive process as it occurs throughout the alimentary canal.

• Describe the mechanical and chemical processes utilized in digestion.

• Discuss the roles of the pancreas and liver in aiding the digestive process.

• Identify the various secretions, enzymes, and hormones used in digestion.

## III. Digestion of Nutrients

### A. Introduction
1.  Digestion is the process of changes that food undergoes in the digestive tract
2.  These changes prepare foods for use by body cells
3.  The types of digestive processes include mechanical digestion and chemical digestion
4.  Mechanical digestion consists of muscle contraction and interaction
    a.  General muscle tone or tonic contractions ensure continuous passage of food mass
    b.  Periodic, rhythmic muscular contraction and relaxation mix and propel the food mass forward
    c.  Alternating muscular contraction and relaxation of the sphincters regulate food movement and prevent reflux into the previous segment
5.  Mechanical digestion is regulated by the nervous system
    a.  Controls muscle tone of the walls of the alimentary canal
    b.  Regulates the rate and intensity of periodic muscle contractions
    c.  Coordinates muscular movements in the digestive tract
6.  Chemical digestion involves the action of specific substances on ingested food; these substances are secreted from specialized cells and glands
    a.  Salivary glands secrete saliva, which contains salivary amylase
    b.  Gastric glands secrete hydrochloric acid and enzymes
    c.  Mucosa or goblet cells secrete mucus directly into the lumen of the digestive tract
    d.  Endocrine and exocrine glands secrete hormones and pancreatic juices
    e.  Multicellular tubular glands secrete intestinal juice
    f.  Liver secretes bile
7.  Chemical digestion is stimulated by:
    a.  Presence of food in a specific segment of the digestive tract
    b.  Parasympathetic and sympathetic innervation
    c.  Digestive hormones specific for certain substances

### B. Mouth and esophagus
1.  Mechanical digestion
    a.  Mastication occurs in the buccal cavity
    b.  Swallowing propels food from the mouth toward the stomach
2.  Chemical digestion
    a.  Secretion of ptyalin in saliva from salivary glands partially digests starches; this action is terminated by the acid pH of the stomach
    b.  Secretion of mucous material from salivary glands lubricates and binds food particles
    c.  Secretion of mucus from mucous glands in esophagus aids in swallowing and forward movement of food mass

**C. Stomach**
   1. Mechanical digestion
      a. Muscles in the stomach stretch outward to hold up to 1 liter of food mass
      b. Local tonic muscle contractions and peristaltic waves mix the food mass and reduce it to chyme
      c. Each peristaltic wave controls emptying of stomach by allowing small amounts of acid chyme through the pyloric valve into the duodenum
   2. Chemical digestion
      a. Secretion of pepsinogen by chief cells helps form pepsin for the breakdown of proteins to smaller polypeptides
      b. Secretion of hydrochloric acid by parietal cells aids in converting proteins to polypeptides
      c. Secretion of mucus by the mucous cells protects the gastric mucosa from the highly acid content; gives body and cohesiveness to the food mass
      d. Secretion of secretin counteracts excessive gastric activity by inhibiting hydrochloric acid and pepsin secretion and gastric motility

**D. Small intestine**
   1. Mechanical digestion
      a. Segmentational muscular contractions, longitudinal muscular rotation, and pendular muscular movements mix the food mass
      b. Peristalsis mixes the intestinal juice and chyme and propels it forward
      c. Villi motions assist with movement and allow chyme to come in contact with the surface for absorption
   2. Chemical digestion
      a. Pancreatic amylase converts starch to disaccharides
      b. Lactase converts lactose to glucose and galactose
      c. Sucrase converts sucrose to glucose and fructose
      d. Maltase converts maltose to glucose and glucose (2 molecules of glucose)
      e. Enterokinase converts the inactive proenzyme trypsinogen to the active enzyme trypsin
      f. Trypsin and chymotrypsin from the pancreas break down proteins and polypeptides to dipeptides
      g. Carboxypolypeptidase from the pancreas, secreted into the duodenum, converts polypeptides to amino acids
      h. Aminopeptidase causes release of amino acids from polypeptides and dipeptides
      i. Dipeptidase converts dipeptides to amino acids
      j. Bicarbonate ions from the pancreas neutralize acid chyme emptied from the stomach into the duodenum
      k. Mucus is secreted to protect mucosa from irritation and digestion by acidic gastric juices
      l. Secretin stimulates pancreatic and bile secretions

      m. Cholecystokinin stimulates the gallbladder to contract and release bile into the duodenum
      n. Bile converts fats to emulsified fats
      o. Intestinal lipase and pancreatic lipase convert fats to monoglycerides, diglycerides, glycerol, and fatty acids

## E. Large intestine
   1. Mechanical digestion
      a. Propulsive or mass movements of the intestinal walls mix the mass and move it forward
      b. The defecation reflex is initiated under both voluntary and involuntary control, and feces leave the rectum
   2. No chemical digestion occurs in the large intestine

## Points to Remember

Both mechanical and chemical digestion occur throughout the alimentary canal to alter the character of food and aid its absorption through the intestinal walls.

Mechanical breakdown and mixing of food increase the contact between nutrients and digestive secretions, promoting chemical digestion.

Chemical digestion breaks down carbohydrates into monosaccharides, lipids into fatty acids and glycerides, and proteins into amino acids.

## Glossary

**Defecation**—elimination of wastes and undigested food from the rectum as feces

**Emulsification**—process of breaking down large particles into smaller ones, holding them in suspension

**Motility**—ability to move spontaneously, such as food through the intestines

**Peristalsis**—alternating muscular contraction and relaxation in the alimentary canal to propel food forward

# Absorption of Nutrients

**Learning Objectives**

After studying this section, the reader should be able to:

- Define absorption.

- Identify the mechanisms of absorption.

- List important factors affecting absorption of nutrients.

- Identify where absorption of essential nutrients occurs.

## IV. Absorption of Nutrients

### A. Introduction

1. Absorption refers to the passage of nutrients through intestinal epithelial cells—mainly in the small intestine—into blood and lymph
2. Surface structures involved in absorption include mucosal folds, villi, and microvilli. These combine to give the intestinal mucosa great absorptive capacity
3. Mechanisms of absorption include:
   a. Passive diffusion
   b. Facilitated diffusion
   c. Active transport
   d. Pinocytosis
4. Routes of absorption include:
   a. Through the microvilli into the portal blood circulation
   b. Through the microvilli into the portal lymph circulation
5. Factors affecting the extent of absorption of a nutrient include:
   a. Properties of the nutrient
   b. Nutrient source
   c. Presence of other nutrients in the intestine
   d. Presence of certain food components, such as fiber, in the intestine
   e. Presence of certain drugs in the intestine
   f. Intestinal motility
   g. Other factors unique to the individual, such as disease states
6. Intestinal absorption accounts for approximately 9.9 liters of the average total daily intake of 10 liters
   a. Total intake consists of approximately 1.5 liters of food and 8.5 liters from GI secretions
   b. The small intestine absorbs approximately 9.5 liters; the large intestine, approximately 0.4 liter
   c. The remaining 0.1 liter is eliminated as feces

### B. Small intestine

1. General information
   a. Most nutrient absorption occurs in the small intestine
   b. Different nutrients are absorbed in different areas of the small intestine
2. Nutrients absorbed in the duodenum
   a. Minerals, such as iron, calcium, zinc, and magnesium
   b. Some digested energy nutrients (carbohydrates, fats, and proteins)
   c. Vitamins A and E, folic acid, riboflavin, and thiamin
3. Nutrients absorbed in the jejunum
   a. The major portion of digested energy nutrients
   b. Vitamins A, $B_6$, C, and D
   c. Minerals, such as sodium, potassium, and chloride
   d. Some water

   4.   Nutrients absorbed in the ileum
        a.   Vitamins $B_{12}$ and K
        b.   Minerals, such as sodium, potassium, and chloride
        c.   Small amounts of energy nutrients and vitamins that weren't absorbed in
             the duodenum and jejunum
        d.   Bile salts
        e.   Some water

## C.  Large intestine
   1.   General information
        a.   The large intestine plays only a minor role in nutrient absorption
        b.   Gases produced in the large intestine are partly absorbed, with the
             remainder expelled as flatus
   2.   Nutrients absorbed in the ascending, transverse, and descending colon
        a.   The major portion of water
        b.   Minerals, such as sodium and potassium
        c.   Vitamin K and possibly biotin
   3.   Nutrients absorbed in the rectum: None

## Points to Remember

During absorption, nutrients pass through intestinal epithelial cells into the blood and lymph.

Most nutrient absorption occurs in the small intestine.

Unabsorbed substances are held in the colon for elimination as feces.

## Glossary

**Active transport**—movement of particles from an area of lower concentration across a cell membrane to an area of higher concentration; requires the expenditure of energy and results in an even distribution of particles

**Facilitated diffusion**—process by which carriers aid molecules too large to enter cells by passive diffusion across the cell membrane

**Passive diffusion**—process by which particles move from an area of higher concentration to an area of lower concentration without any expenditure of energy; results in an even distribution of particles

**Pinocytosis**—process by which extracellular fluid is taken into a cell; the cell membrane forms a saccular indentation filled with extracellular fluid and then closes around it to form a vacuole of fluid within the cell

# Water

**Learning Objectives**
After studying this section, the reader should be able to:

● Describe the general characteristics of water as a nutrient.

● Identify the factors affecting water balance.

● List the functions of water as a nutrient.

● Discuss the processes of absorption and metabolism of water.

● State the dietary requirements of water.

● Describe the sources of dietary water.

## V. Water

### A. Introduction

1. Water is the principal constituent of all living organisms and the most abundant component of the human body
2. Water is present in all body tissues and is essential to all biochemical processes, including energy production of adenosine triphosphate (ATP)
3. Water contains no calories
4. Water is an end product of the metabolism of energy-producing nutrients
5. Approximately 50% to 60% of an adult's total body weight (TBW) is water
6. Water in body fluids is contained in fluid compartments; it accounts for approximately 40 liters in a man of average weight (154 lb [70 kg])
   a. Intracellular fluid (ICF) accounts for approximately 25 liters of water; chiefly contained in muscle tissues
   b. Extracellular fluid (ECF) accounts for approximately 15 liters of water; can be further subdivided into intravascular and interstitial fluid compartments
7. Regulators of water intake include:
   a. The thirst center located in the hypothalamus (major regulator)
   b. Antidiuretic hormone (ADH), which causes an increase in renal absorption of water
   c. Aldosterone, which can cause retention of sodium, and therefore water, by the kidneys
8. Water intake must be equivalent to water elimination for homeostasis (see *Intake and output* on page 28 for more information)
9. Water may be eliminated through:
   a. Kidneys, in urine
   b. Skin, in perspiration
   c. Lungs, as expired water vapor
   d. Bowel, in feces
10. Factors affecting body water or fluid balance include:
    a. Age: Up to 75% of a newborn's TBW consists of water; this percentage decreases from birth to old age
    b. Environmental and body temperature: In very hot weather, water loss as perspiration can increase as much as 1.5 to 2.0 liters an hour
    c. Exercise: Water loss through the respiratory tract and through perspiration increases with body heat
    d. Emotional or physical stress (such as anxiety, pain, or fear): Fluid retention increases through the action of ADH
    e. Surgery and anesthetics: Fluid retention increases through the action of ADH
    f. Diseases (such as renal failure, cancer, and hypertension): Fluid retention or fluid output increases through various mechanisms
    g. Trauma (such as burns and crush injuries): Third space fluid may shift and cause fluid imbalance
    h. Drugs (such as diuretics): Fluid loss through the kidneys may increase and body fluids may become imbalanced

## INTAKE AND OUTPUT

| DAILY INTAKE | | DAILY OUTPUT | |
| --- | --- | --- | --- |
| Liquids | 1,400 ml | Kidneys (urine) | 1,500 ml |
| Liquids in foods | 700 ml | Skin | 350 ml |
| Metabolism of foods | 300 ml | Lungs (water vapor) | 400 ml |
| | | Intestines (feces) | 150 ml |
| Total intake | 2,400 ml | Total output | 2,400 ml |

**B. Functions**
1. Provides an aqueous medium for all body fluids, secretions, and excretions, such as blood, lymph, urine, and perspiration
2. Transports nutrients to cells
3. Transports wastes away from cells
4. Provides a medium for excretion of wastes from the body
5. Aids in digestion of foods through hydrolysis
6. Regulates body temperature through insensible water loss from the skin
7. Maintains the physical and chemical constancy of such body fluids as plasma and lymph
8. Acts as a lubricant in the pleural cavity and pericardium

**C. Digestion:** No digestion of water is necessary

**D. Metabolism and absorption**
1. Water is an end product of metabolism from the energy-producing nutrients: carbohydrates, lipids, and proteins
2. Water is transported freely in both directions across the intestinal mucosa
3. Approximately 7 to 8 liters are reabsorbed in the small intestine daily
4. Approximately 100 ml daily remain in the digestive tract for excretion in the feces

**E. Dietary requirements**
1. No specific intake requirements have been established other than to maintain a balance of fluid intake and output
2. Researchers suggest three 8-oz glasses of water daily in addition to other beverages

**F. Sources**
1. By drinking fluids; accounts for approximately 1,300 to 1,500 ml/day
2. Through the liquid component of foods ingested; accounts for approximately 700 to 1,000 ml/day
3. From water produced when nutrients are oxidized during metabolism; accounts for approximately 200 to 300 ml/day

## Points to Remember

Water is essential to maintain fluid balance within the body.

Water is the principal constituent of all living organisms.

The amount of water in the body is determined by the balance between fluid intake and fluid output.

## Glossary

**Extracellular fluid**—fluid outside the cell

**Homeostasis**—state of internal equilibrium maintained by feedback and regulatory processes

**Hydrolysis**—chemical breakdown of food into simpler substances through reaction with water

**Interstitial fluid**—fluid in the tissues

**Intracellular fluid**—fluid within the cell

**Intravascular fluid**—fluid within a vessel

**Osmosis**—movement of solvent, most often water, through a semipermeable membrane from an area of lower solute concentration to an area of higher solute concentration, equalizing the concentrations

# Carbohydrates

**Learning Objectives**

After studying this section, the reader should be able to:

- Describe the general characteristics of carbohydrates.

- List the functions of carbohydrates.

- Describe the classification of carbohydrates.

- Discuss the process of digestion of carbohydrates.

- State the dietary requirements for carbohydrates.

- Identify the dietary sources for carbohydrates.

# VI. Carbohydrates

## A. Introduction
1. Carbohydrates are essential nutrients composed of carbon, hydrogen, and oxygen
2. Obtained primarily from plant sources, carbohydrates are the cheapest, most easily obtainable nutrient and the most readily digested form of fuel for the body
3. In the United States, carbohydrates constitute about 45% of the average diet

## B. Functions
1. Provide energy
   a. Yield 4 calories per gram
   b. Are the most readily available source of energy for the body
   c. Can be stored and released when the body needs energy
   d. Are the only energy source used by the central nervous system under normal conditions
   e. Are the only energy source used by the lens of the eye
2. Provide nutrient-sparing action
   a. Prevent excessive oxidation of fats for energy
   b. Prevent muscle wasting; because carbohydrates are used first for energy production, they spare protein for protein synthesis
3. Regulate GI functions
   a. Fermentation of dietary lactose encourages growth of normal bacterial flora and discourages growth of undesirable bacterial flora
   b. Absorption of water by dietary fiber retards gastric emptying and aids fermentation by intestinal bacteria

## C. Classification
1. Monosaccharides
   a. These simplest carbohydrates cannot be broken down further
   b. Major monosaccharides include *glucose, fructose,* and *galactose*
   c. Glucose, also known as dextrose and corn syrup, is the main source of energy for cells. It's the principal product of digestion of disaccharides and polysaccharides
   d. Fructose, also known as levulose, is the sweetest of the monosaccharides and one of the end products of sucrose digestion
   e. Galactose is not found free in nature, and is one of the end products of lactose digestion
2. Disaccharides
   a. Disaccharides are composed of two monosaccharides
   b. Major dissacharides include *sucrose, lactose,* and *maltose*
   c. Sucrose, also known as invert sugar, is broken down into glucose and fructose
   d. Lactose, also known as milk sugar, is broken down into glucose and galactose

     e. Maltose, or malt sugar, is broken down into glucose and glucose (2 molecules of glucose)

3. Polysaccharides
   a. Polysaccharides are complex carbohydrates made up of multiple monosaccharides
   b. Major polysaccharides include *starch, glycogen* (stored carbohydrates), *cellulose,* and *hemicellulose*
   c. Starch, the most abundant source of dietary carbohydrates, is reduced to glucose through a complex enzymatic process
   d. Glycogen is stored in the liver and muscles as a form of stored energy
   e. Cellulose, an indigestible fiber also known as dietary fiber, bulk, or roughage, promotes efficient intestinal function
   f. Hemicellulose, also known as bran, is an indigestible grain fiber

**D. Digestion**
1. General information
   a. Monosaccharides require no digestion
   b. Disaccharides and polysaccharides are broken down into monosaccharides by digestive enzymes
   c. Glucose is the most important end product of carbohydrate digestion
   d. Salivary amylase in the mouth initiates the breakdown of starch into starch dextrins
2. Stomach
   a. No specific digestion of carbohydrates occurs in the stomach
   b. Hydrolysis of starch dextrins continues
3. Small intestine
   a. Pancreatic amylase further breaks down starch dextrins into maltose
   b. Sucrase breaks down sucrose into glucose and fructose
   c. Lactase breaks down lactose into glucose and galactose
   d. Maltase breaks down maltose into glucose and glucose (2 molecules of glucose)

**E. Metabolism and absorption**
1. Absorption occurs by active transport through the small intestinal mucosa
2. Rate of absorption depends on:
   a. Speed that carbohydrates are released into small intestine
   b. Mixture of food present in intestine
   c. Hormones present
3. Glucose is catabolized to release energy (glycolysis); end products of carbohydrate metabolism are energy, carbon dioxide, and water
4. Excess glucose intake is anabolized into glycogen for storage (glycogenesis); may be broken down to release energy (glycogenolysis)
5. Glucose is converted to fats and stored in adipose tissue after glycogen stores are filled

**F.  Dietary requirements**
1.  Specific requirements for carbohydrates have not been established
2.  Adults should consume 50 to 100 grams of carbohydrates daily to prevent ketosis
3.  Approximately 55% of daily calories should be ingested as carbohydrates; most of these should be in the form of complex carbohydrates
4.  Between 15 to 20 grams of dietary fiber should be included in total daily intake

**G.  Sources**
1.  Grain products
    a.  Cereals
    b.  Flours and breads
    c.  Pasta
2.  Fruits, such as apples, oranges, and prunes
3.  Vegetables, such as corn, potatoes, dried beans, and peas
4.  Milk and other dairy products
5.  Refined sugars and concentrated sweets, such as white sugar, brown sugar, confectioners sugar, honey, and maple syrup

## Points to Remember

Dietary carbohydrates include simple sugars, starches, and dietary fiber.

Dietary carbohydrates are broken down into monosaccharides in the digestive tract and converted to glucose in the liver.

Although no set dietary requirements have been established for carbohydrates, they should be supplied in the daily diet to prevent ketosis and muscle wasting.

## Glossary

**Complex carbohydrates**—carbohydrates formed by many monosaccharides

**Fermentation**—decomposition of an organic substance into simpler compounds

**Glycolysis**—breakdown of glucose to provide energy

**Ketosis**—accumulation of by-products of fat metabolism in the blood

**Oxidation**—process of combining or causing a substance to combine with oxygen

# Lipids

**Learning Objectives**

After studying this section, the reader should be able to:

- Describe the general characteristics of lipids.

- List the functions of lipids.

- Describe the classifications of lipids.

- Discuss the process of digestion of lipids.

- State the dietary requirements of lipids.

- Identify the dietary sources for lipids.

## VII. Lipids

### A. Introduction

1. Lipids are essential nutrients containing carbon, hydrogen, and oxygen
2. They are relatively insoluble in water but soluble in such organic solvents as ether and chloroform
3. They provide a concentrated form of energy, yielding 9 calories per gram
4. They are stored compactly with little or no water in adipose tissue and can be directly oxidized for energy
5. Lipids account for 35% to 45% of the total daily caloric intake in the average American diet
6. Lipids can be grouped according to structure. The fundamental structural unit is a fatty acid consisting of a chain or string of carbon molecules
   a. Short-chain fatty acids (SCFAs) contain between 2 and 6 carbons
   b. Medium-chain fatty acids (MCFAs) contain between 8 and 12 carbons
   c. Long-chain fatty acids (LCFAs) contain between 14 and 24 carbons
7. Essential fatty acids (EFAs) cannot be synthesized by the body and must be supplied in the diet; they include:
   a. Linoleic acid
   b. Linolenic acid
   c. Arachidonic acid (Because it can be synthesized in the body from linoleic acid, some sources do not list it as an EFA)
8. Lipids may be classified chemically as simple, compound, or derived
9. Simple lipids are esters of glycerol and fatty acids
   a. Glycerol is a water-soluble alcohol that forms an ester when combined with an acid and can be used by the body to make glucose
   b. Simple lipids can be classified as monoglycerides, diglycerides, and triglycerides
   c. Triglycerides, the most common lipid, account for approximately 98% of the lipids found in foods and 90% of the lipids in the body
10. Compound lipids are combinations of simple lipids with nonlipid substances
    a. Examples include phospholipids, simple lipids combined with phosphorus; glycolipids, simple lipids combined with glucose; and lipoproteins, simple lipids combined with a plasma protein
    b. Lipoproteins are synthenized in the liver and are the form in which lipids circulate in the blood
11. Derived lipids are substances produced during the breakdown of simple and compound lipids
    a. Examples include cholesterol, steroid hormones, and ergosterol
    b. Cholesterol functions as an essential component of brain and nervous tissues, a precursor of vitamin D and steroid hormones, a constituent of bile salts, and a structural component of cell membranes
    c. Increased serum cholesterol levels are associated with atherosclerosis

**B.  Functions**
   1.  Supply a continuous source of fuel for the body to use or store as needed
   2.  Supply essential fatty acids
   3.  Contribute to the taste and flavor of foods
   4.  Contribute to the feeling of satiety after eating
   5.  Spare protein for protein synthesis rather than for energy production
   6.  Allow proper absorption of fat-soluble vitamins

**C.  Classification**
   1.  The degree of saturation of a lipid refers to its atomic structure and is determined by the number of hydrogen atoms present; hydrogen atoms bond to carbon atoms, and the greater the number of bonded hydrogen atoms, the more saturated the molecule
   2.  Saturated fatty acids
       a.  Have all carbon atoms bound to hydrogen atoms
       b.  Are solid at room temperature
       c.  Are linked to elevated serum cholesterol levels and atherosclerosis
       d.  Include palmitic and stearic acids
   3.  Unsaturated fatty acids
       a.  Have carbon atoms available for hydrogen atom bonding
       b.  Are usually liquid at room temperature
       c.  Are divided into monounsaturated and polyunsaturated fatty acids; monounsaturated fatty acids can only bind with one additional hydrogen atom, whereas polyunsaturated fatty acids can bind with two or more hydrogen atoms
       d.  Oleic acid is the most abundant monounsaturated fatty acid
       e.  Plant fats are predominantly polyunsaturated fatty acids
       f.  Polyunsaturated fatty acids include linoleic, linolenic, and arachidonic acids

**D.  Digestion**
   1.  General information
       a.  Fats remain in the stomach up to 3½ hours after ingestion
       b.  SCFAs and MCFAs are digested to the same degree as are other water-soluble substances
       c.  LCFAs are digested to a greater extent
   2.  Mouth: The chewing process physically breaks down LCFAs and warms them
   3.  Stomach
       a.  Gastric lipase begins chemical hydrolysis of LCFAs
       b.  Fat in the chyme stimulates release of cholecystokinin, which stimulates the gallbladder to release bile
       c.  Bile salts emulsify and reduce the surface tension of fats, which are then divided into smaller particles

4.  Pancreas and intestines
    a.  Peristalsis facilitates the mixing and emulsification process by bile
    b.  Lipase in pancreatic and intestinal secretions hydrolyze triglycerides to fatty acids and glycerol

**E.  Metabolism and absorption**
1.  SCFAs, MCFAs, and glycerol are absorbed directly into the bloodstream, then carried to the liver and stored
2.  LCFAs are changed into a form that can be carried through the blood and absorbed through the walls of the small intestine; they then enter the bloodstream through the lymphatic system
3.  About 97% of fat is absorbed, with the remainder eliminated in the feces
4.  Lipid metabolism occurs mainly in the liver. Processes include:
    a.  Synthesis of triglycerides from carbohydrates and some proteins
    b.  Synthesis of other lipids, such as phospholipids and cholesterol, from triglycerides
    c.  Desaturation of fatty acids
    d.  Degradation of triglycerides for use as energy
5.  Hormones play a role in fat metabolism, facilitating the release of fatty acids from adipose tissue
6.  End products of fat metabolism include fatty acids and glycerol

**F.  Dietary requirements**
1.  Specific requirements for fats have not been established
2.  Fats must be supplied by the diet; estimated required daily intake is approximately 2% of daily calories
3.  American Heart Association (AHA) guidelines recommend reducing total daily fat intake to approximately 30% of daily calories
4.  The AHA also recommends a total daily cholesterol intake below 300 mg (See Section XI, Dietary Guidelines, for more AHA guidelines)
5.  Recommendations for health problems related to dietary fat intake focus on intake of total fat and of saturated fat

**G.  Sources**
1.  Animal sources that are high in fat include lard, butter, beef, lamb, pork, egg yolks, cheese, milk, and cream
2.  Vegetable sources that are high in fat include vegetables oils, nuts, seeds, chocolate, olives, and avocados

## Points to Remember

Fats vary greatly in their physical and chemical properties, depending on their fatty acids.

Because of their insolubility in water, fats require special conditions for digestion, absorption, and transportation in the body.

Recommendations for health problems related to dietary fat intake focus on two main issues: excessive total fat intake and saturated fat intake.

## Glossary

**Atherosclerosis**—characterized by degeneration and hardening of the arteries and sometimes the valves of the heart

**Degradation**—process of breaking down a substance into a less complex form

**Desaturation**—process of converting a saturated compound into an unsaturated one by releasing bonded hydrogen atoms

**Ester**—compound formed from an alcohol and an acid by removing water

**Lipoprotein**—combination of a lipid and a protein, having the general properties of proteins

# Proteins

## Learning Objectives

After studying this section, the reader should be able to:

- Describe the general characteristics of proteins.

- Discuss nitrogen balance and the role of proteins.

- List the functions of proteins.

- Describe the classifications of amino acids.

- Identify the essential amino acids.

- Discuss the process of digestion of proteins.

- State the dietary requirements of proteins.

- Identify the dietary sources for proteins.

# VIII. Proteins

## A. Introduction

1. Proteins are organic substances containing carbon, hydrogen, oxygen, and nitrogen; they are the only energy-producing nutrient to contain nitrogen and thus the only nutrient to have nitrogen as a waste product of metabolism
2. Proteins consist of large molecular structures that do not readily pass through cell membranes
3. Adequate protein is necessary for maintenance of body tissue; increased protein is necessary to support growth
4. An essential nutrient, proteins are the most plentiful substance in the body next to water, present in every living cell and constituting about 75% of body solids
5. They are contained in muscle, bone, cartilage, skin, blood, and lymph and form the components of many hormones and all enzymes
6. As much as 95% of ingested protein is broken down into amino acids
7. Proteins exist as simple or compound forms
   a. Simple proteins contain only amino acids or their derivatives and include albumin, globulin, glutelin, and prolamin
   b. Compound or conjugated proteins contain a simple protein and another nonprotein group and include hemoglobin, mucin, cholesterol, and purines
8. Proteins are the body's only source of dietary nitrogen
9. The body's nitrogen balance is a direct indication of the body's protein status
   a. In nitrogen equilibrium, nitrogen intake equals nitrogen excretion, as in the normal state of tissue maintenance
   b. In positive nitrogen balance—an increase in body protein—nitrogen intake exceeds nitrogen excretion, as happens in growth and other anabolic states
   c. In negative nitrogen balance—a decrease in body protein—nitrogen excretion exceeds nitrogen intake, as happens when the body uses protein as an energy source

## B. Functions

1. Furnish amino acids necessary for building and repairing body tissue
2. Contribute to the formation of essential body secretions and fluids, including enzymes, mucus, antibodies, hormones, and hemoglobin
3. Aid in the regulation of acid-base balance by acting as buffers
4. Control the osmotic pressure between body fluids (plasma proteins)
5. Function in the transport of other substances; for example, lipids are transported as lipoproteins and albumin transports free fatty acids and bilirubin
6. Provide a source of energy (4 calories per gram) when carbohydrates and fats are inadequate

7.  Furnish amino acids, such as tryptophan and histidine, needed to make compounds used in metabolic functions
8.  Contribute to the production of immunoglobulins that increase disease resistance

C. **Classification of amino acids**
1.  Essential amino acids (EAAs)
    a.  EAAs must be provided by diet; all must be present simultaneously to be used by the body
    b.  EAAs cannot be synthesized by the body
    c.  EAAs are needed for tissue growth and maintenance
    d.  The eight EAAs are isoleucine, leucine, lysine, methionine, phenylalanine, threonine, tryptophan, and valine
    e.  Foods that contain the eight EAAs in adequate amounts are called *complete proteins*; these include most animal proteins, including meat, dairy products, fish, poultry, and eggs
    f.  Foods that do not contain the eight EAAs or contain them in insufficient amounts are called *incomplete proteins*; these include cereals, legumes, and vegetables
2.  Semiessential amino acids (SEAAs)
    a.  SEAAs are needed for tissue growth and maintenance in children
    b.  SEAAs cannot be synthesized in a child's body in sufficient quantity to support growth
    c.  SEAAs include arginine and histidine
3.  Nonessential amino acids (NEAAs)
    a.  NEAAs need not be provided by diet
    b.  NEAAs can be synthesized in the liver from other amino acids
    c.  NEAAs include alanine, asparagine, aspartic acid, cystine, glutamic acid, glutamine, glycine, hydroxyproline, hydroxylysine, proline, serine, and tryosine

D. **Digestion**
1.  General information
    a.  Proteins must be broken down into amino acids to be absorbed
    b.  Digestion of amino acids is slow
2.  Mouth: Mechanical action breaks down protein foods into smaller pieces
3.  Stomach
    a.  Hydrochloric acid converts the inactive enzyme pepsinogen to the active enzyme pepsin, which breaks down protein into smaller polypeptides
    b.  Rennin breaks down casein (milk protein) and readies it for the action of pepsin; this process is necessary for the digestion of milk by infants
4.  Small intestine
    a.  Pancreatic secretions: trypsin and chymotrypsin further break down polypeptides to dipeptides; carboxypeptidase converts polypeptides to amino acids

b. Intestinal secretions: aminopeptidase breaks down polypeptides and dipeptides to amino acids; dipeptidase breaks down dipeptides to amino acids

## E. Metabolism and absorption

1. Proteins are absorbed as amino acids through the small intestine directly into portal circulation
2. Absorption occurs rapidly; requires energy, vitamin $B_6$, and manganese
3. Amino acids are transported to cells by active transport and facilitated diffusion
4. End products of protein metabolism consist of amino acids
5. Protein *anabolism* occurs in all body cells
   a. Anabolism is influenced by EAAs, caloric intake, and hormones, including growth hormone, androgens, estrogens, thyroxine, and insulin
   b. Types of protein formed depend on functional and genetic characteristics of the cell
6. Protein *catabolism* occurs to limit the amount of protein that can accumulate in a cell; it is affected by certain hormones, such as adrenocorticoids, glucagon, and thyroxine
7. Additional amino acids are degraded by the process of *deamination*
   a. The amino group ($NH_2$) of the amino acid is hydrolyzed and combines with water from hydrolysis to form ammonia
   b. Ammonia is removed from blood, transported to the liver, and converted to urea for excretion by the kidneys
   c. Keto acids, the end products of deamination, may be oxidized to release energy through the Krebs cycle, be used to make NEAAs, or be converted to fats and stored as fatty tissue
8. End products of protein catabolism include urea, creatinine, uric acid, and ammonia salts
9. Approximately 75% of ingested nitrogen is eliminated, principally in the urine

## F. Dietary requirements

1. Recommendations for dietary protein intake are based on age and approximate weight
2. In general, protein intake should not exceed 15% to 20% of the total daily caloric intake
3. See Appendix A for specific recommended dietary allowances (RDAs)

## G. Sources

1. Complete proteins, such as whole milk, lean meat, cottage cheese, eggs, fish, poultry
2. Incomplete proteins, such as beans, peas, corn, wheat bread

## Points to Remember

Proteins, made up of amino acids, are required in adequate amounts for the constant replacement of body tissues, with additional amounts needed to support growth.

Protein is the only energy-producing nutrient to contain nitrogen and thus the only one to have nitrogen as a waste product of metabolism.

All the essential amino acids must be present at the same time for adequate protein use by the body.

The body uses protein as an energy source only if sufficient calories for energy requirements are not available from carbohydrates or fats.

## Glossary

**Acid-base balance**—maintenance of a normal equilibirum between the acidity and alkalinity of body fluids

**Deamination**—breaking down of amino acids

**Hemoglobin**—a conjugated protein that contains four heme groups and globin; transports oxygen to cells

**Immunoglobulins**—antibodies; the body's main protection from infection

**Organic substance**—any substance that contains carbon; pertains to substances derived from living organisms

# Vitamins

**Learning Objectives**

After studying this section, the reader should be able to:

- Describe the general characteristics of vitamins.

- List the functions of the specific vitamins.

- Describe the classifications of vitamins.

- State the dietary requirements for the specific vitamins.

- Identify the dietary sources for the specific vitamins.

- Identify the clinical manifestations of specific vitamin deficiencies.

- Identify the clinical manifestations of major vitamin toxicities.

## IX. Vitamins

### A. Introduction
1. Vitamins are organic compounds containing carbon, hydrogen, and, in some cases, oxygen, nitrogen, and sulfur
2. Required in minute amounts for growth, maintenance, and repair of body tissues, vitamins also help regulate metabolism and act as catalysts in biochemical reactions
3. Vitamins aren't produced by the body, but must be supplied through diet or dietary supplements
4. They are destroyed readily by heat, oxidation, and certain chemical processes
5. Vitamin requirements increase during periods of stress

### B. Functions: Each vitamin has its own specific functions; see *Vitamins* for more information

### C. Classification
1. Fat-soluble vitamins
   a. Soluble in fat or fat solvents
   b. Fairly stable when heated
   c. Do not contain nitrogen
   d. Absorbed in small intestine with fats in food
   e. Require bile salts for absorption
   f. Can be stored in body to some extent
   g. Normally are not excreted in urine
   h. Provided by dietary intake; daily intake not required
   i. May have decreased absorption with certain conditions, such as fat malabsorption and antibiotic therapy
   j. Include vitamins A, D, E, and K
2. Water-soluble vitamins
   a. Not stored in body in adequate amounts
   b. Must be provided daily through dietary intake
   c. Excess amounts excreted in urine
   d. Include vitamins C, $B_1$, $B_2$, $B_6$, and $B_{12}$, and folic acid, niacin, biotin, and pantothenic acid; the B vitamins contain nitrogen

### D. Digestion: Vitamins are not digested, but are used in their ingested form

### E. Metabolism, absorption, storage, elimination
1. Vitamin absorption occurs in the small intestine
2. No metabolism occurs

## VITAMINS

| MAIN FOOD SOURCES | MAJOR FUNCTIONS | DEFICIENCY AND TOXICITY FINDINGS |
|---|---|---|
| **Water-soluble vitamins*** | | |
| **VITAMIN C (ascorbic acid)** | | |
| Fresh fruits (especially citrus) and vegetables | Collagen formation, bone and tooth formation, iodine conservation, healing, red blood cell formation, infection resistance, iron absorption and use, corticosteroid synthesis | *Deficiency (Scurvy):* bleeding gums, easy bruising, dyspnea, low infection resistance, nosebleeds, tooth decay, anorexia, fatigue, irritability, muscle and joint pain, skin lesions<br>*Toxicity* (rare): GI upset, impaired leukocyte bactericidal activity, excessive iron absorption, uricosuria with resultant renal calculi, pancreatic damage resulting in decreased insulin production |
| **VITAMIN B₁ (thiamine)** | | |
| Meats, fish, poultry, pork, molasses, brewer's yeast, brown rice, nuts, wheat germ, whole and enriched grains | Carbohydrate, fat, protein metabolism; energy production; central nervous system maintenance | *Deficiency (Beriberi):* weakness, appetite loss, constipation, dyspnea, fatigue, irritability, memory loss, myocardial pain, nervousness, hand and foot numbness, pain and noise sensitivity, ataxia<br>*Toxicity:* Edema, sweating, tremors, tachycardia, hypotension |
| **VITAMIN B₂ (riboflavin)** | | |
| Meats, fish, poultry, milk, molasses, brewer's yeast, eggs, fruit, green leafy vegetables, nuts, whole grains | Antibody and red blood cell formation; energy production; epithelial, eye, and mucosal tissue maintenance | *Deficiency:* Cataracts, cheilosis, dizziness, eye fatigue, itching and burning eyes, light sensitivity, oily skin, retarded growth, tongue redness and soreness<br>*Toxicity:* No known effects |
| **VITAMIN B₆ (pyridoxine)** | | |
| Meats, poultry, bananas, molasses, brewer's yeast, desiccated liver, fish, green leafy vegetables, peanuts, raisins, walnuts, wheat germ, whole grains | Antibody formation, digestion, DNA and RNA synthesis, fat and protein metabolism, hemoglobin production, sodium and potassium balance, central nervous system maintenance, tryptophan to niacin conversion | *Deficiency:* Seborrheic dermatitis, acne, arthritis, glossitis, cheilosis, seizures (in infants), depression, dizziness, hair loss, irritability, learning disabilities, ataxia, weakness<br>*Toxicity* (rare): Occurs only with 3 g/kg dose |
| **FOLIC ACID (folacin; pteroylglutamic acid)** | | |
| Citrus fruits, eggs, green leafy vegetables, milk products, organ meats, seafood, whole grains | Red and white blood cell formation and maturation, DNA and RNA formation | *Deficiency:* Macrocytic or megaloblastic anemia, fatigue, weakness, fainting, pallor, digestive problems, graying hair, growth problems, insomnia, tongue inflammation, memory impairment<br>*Toxicity:* No known effects |

continued

*For specific RDAs of each vitamin, see Appendix A.

**VITAMINS** continued

| MAIN FOOD SOURCES | MAJOR FUNCTIONS | DEFICIENCY AND TOXICITY FINDINGS |
|---|---|---|
| NIACIN (nicotinic acid, nicotinamide, niacinamide) | | |
| Eggs, lean meats, milk products, organ meats, peanuts, poultry, seafood, whole grains | Cholesterol level reduction, metabolism (carbohydrate, protein, fat), sex hormone production, glycogen synthesis | *Deficiency:* Diarrhea, depression, appetite loss, canker sores, fatigue, halitosis, headaches, indigestion, insomnia, memory impairment, muscle weakness, nausea, nervous disorders, skin eruptions, pellagra (symmetrical dermatitis) <br> *Toxicity:* Flushing, vasodilation (only with large nicotinic acid doses) |
| VITAMIN $B_{12}$ (cyanocobalamin) | | |
| Beef, eggs, fish, milk products, organ meats, pork | Red blood cell maturation, cellular and nutrient metabolism, cell longevity, iron absorption, tissue growth, nerve cell maintenance, myelin formation | *Deficiency* (most common in vegetarians): Fatigue, memory impairment, mental depression and confusion, nervousness, reduced reflex responses, walking and speech problems, glossitis, headache, pernicious anemia <br> *Toxicity:* No known effects |
| BIOTIN | | |
| Egg yolks, legumes, organ meats, whole grains, yeast, milk, seafood, vegetables | Cell growth; fatty acid synthesis, metabolism (carbohydrate, fat, protein), vitamin B use, energy production | *Deficiency:* Depression, dry skin, anemia, glossitis, insomnia, muscle pain, anorexia <br> *Toxicity:* No known effects |
| PANTOTHENIC ACID (formerly called vitamin $B_3$) | | |
| Eggs, legumes, mushrooms, organ meats, salmon, wheat germ, whole grains, fresh vegetables, yeast | Antibody formation, metabolism (carbohydrates, fats, and protein), cortisone production, growth stimulation, stress tolerance, cholesterol synthesis | *Deficiency* (rare): Diarrhea, eczema, hair loss, muscle cramps, nervousness, premature aging, respiratory infections, fatigue, numbness <br> *Toxicity:* No known effects |
| **Fat-soluble vitamins*** | | |
| VITAMIN A (retinol, provitamin A) | | |
| Fish, green and yellow fruits and vegetables, milk products | Body tissue repair and maintenance, infection resistance, bone growth, nervous system development, cell membrane metabolism and structure, RNA synthesis, visual purple production (for night vision) | *Deficiency:* Allergies; appetite loss; dry hair; fatigue; frequent ear, mouth, or salivary gland infections; itching and burning eyes; loss of smell; night blindness; rough, dry, scaly skin; sinus problems; softened tooth enamel <br> *Toxicity:* Skin dryness and desquamation, hair loss, bone pain and fragility, enlarged liver and spleen, headache, pruritus, clubbing of fingers |

**VITAMINS** continued

| MAIN FOOD SOURCES | MAJOR FUNCTIONS | DEFICIENCY AND TOXICITY FINDINGS |
|---|---|---|
| VITAMIN D (calciferol; subtypes include $D_2$ [ergocalciferol] and $D_3$ [cholecalciferol]) | | |
| Bone meal, egg yolks, organ meats, butter, cod liver oil, fatty fish | Calcium and phosphorus use, mineralization of bones and teeth, serum calcium level regulation | *Deficiency:* Burning sensation in mouth and throat, diarrhea, insomnia, myopia, nervousness, softened bones and teeth, rickets (in infants and children), osteomalacia (in adults) *Toxicity:* Polyuria, nocturia, weight loss, muscle weakness, headache, nausea, vomiting, diarrhea, bloody stools, loss of appetite. With *severe* toxicity, soft tissue calcification |
| VITAMIN E (tocopherol) | | |
| Butter, dark green vegetables, eggs, fruits, nuts, organ meats, vegetable oils, whole grains | Cell membrane protection, RBC hemolysis prevention, sexual potency and fertility maintenance (unproved) | *Deficiency:* Edema and skin lesions in infants, anemia, RBC hemolysis, dry or dull hair, hair loss, muscle wasting *Toxicity:* Bleeding, disturbed vitamin A and K utilization, skeletal muscle weakness, GI upset |
| VITAMIN K (menadione; subtypes include $K_2$ [menaquinone] and $K_3$) | | |
| Green leafy vegetables, safflower oil, yogurt, liver, molasses | Liver synthesis of prothrombin and other blood clotting factors | *Deficiency* (rare): Hemorrhagic tendency, miscarriage, nosebleeds *Toxicity* (most common in infants): Kernicterus |

*For specific RDAs of each vitamin, see Appendix A.

3. Fat-soluble vitamins are stored in limited amounts and released to meet the body's needs when intake is inadequate
4. Water-soluble vitamins are not stored; excess amounts are eliminated in urine

F. **Dietary requirements:** See Appendix A for recommended dietary allowances (RDAs) for specific vitamins

G. **Sources:** See *Vitamins,* pages 47 to 49, for specific information

H. **Deficiency and toxicity findings:** See *Vitamins,* pages 47 to 49, for specific information

## Points to Remember

Vitamins are chemically dissimilar organic compounds required by the body in minute amounts for growth, maintenance, and repair of body tissue.

Vitamins are grouped on the basis of solubility. Fat-soluble vitamins include vitamins A, D, E, and K; water-soluble vitamins include the B-complex vitamins and vitamin C.

Vitamins are absorbed but not metabolized; unused fat-soluble vitamins are stored in the body, whereas unused water-soluble vitamins are eliminated in urine.

## Glossary

**Catalyst**—substance that either speeds or slows a chemical reaction

**Deficiency**—condition resulting from the lack of one or more essential nutrients

**Toxicity**—condition resulting from exposure to poisonous amounts of one or more of the vitamins or minerals

# Minerals

**Learning Objectives**

After studying this section, the reader should be able to:

• Describe the general characteristics of minerals.

• List the functions of minerals.

• Describe the classification of minerals.

• Discuss the process of digestion of minerals.

• State the dietary requirements for the various minerals.

• Identify the dietary sources for the various minerals.

• Identify the clinical manifestations of specific mineral deficiencies.

• Identify the clinical manifestations of major mineral toxicities.

## X. Minerals

### A. Introduction

1. Minerals exist only in nature and are not manufactured by the body
2. Minerals exist in two forms: *nonmetallic* elements, consisting of organic substances, and *metallic* elements, consisting of inorganic substances
3. Minerals constitute 60% to 90% of all the inorganic material in the body
4. Minerals in their inorganic form can be supplied in sufficient amounts by an adequate diet, but they must be broken down into their ionic form to be used by the body

### B. Functions: For details about each mineral, see *Minerals*

1. Help regulate enzyme metabolism
2. Help maintain acid-base balance and osmotic pressure
3. Maintain nerve and muscle integrity
4. Facilitate membrane transfer of essential compounds
5. Contribute indirectly to tissue growth
6. Form the components of important body structures, such as bones and teeth

### C. Classification

1. Major elements
   a. Also called macronutrients, macroelements, or macrominerals
   b. Require daily intake greater than 100 mg
   c. Include calcium, chloride, magnesium, phosphorus, potassium, sodium and sulfur
2. Major trace elements
   a. Also called micronutrients, microelements, or microminerals
   b. Require daily intake less than 100 mg
   c. Include chromium, cobalt, copper, fluorine, iodine, iron, manganese, molybdenum, selenium, and zinc
3. Other trace elements
   a. Found in the body in minute amounts
   b. Physiologic roles and sources not identified
   c. Not known if essential to health
   d. Have been used therapeutically
   e. Include aluminum, arsenic, boron, cadmium, nickel, silicon, tin, and vanadium

### D. Digestion

1. The rate of digestion varies among minerals
2. Digestion breaks down the mineral into its ionic form for use by the body

### E. Metabolism, absorption, storage, and elimination

1. Rates of absorption and metabolism vary among minerals
2. Absorption usually occurs in the small intestine
3. Unabsorbed minerals are eliminated in either urine or feces

## MINERALS

| MAIN FOOD SOURCES | MAJOR FUNCTIONS | DEFICIENCY AND TOXICITY FINDINGS |
|---|---|---|
| **Major Elements** | | |
| **CALCIUM*** | | |
| Bonemeal, cheese, milk, molasses, yogurt, whole grains, nuts, legumes, leafy vegetables | Blood clotting, bone and tooth formation, cardiac rhythm regulation, cell membrane structure and function, muscle growth and contraction, nerve impulse transmission | *Deficiency* (hypocalcemia): Paresthesias, heart palpitations, irritability, insomnia, muscle cramps, tetany, Chvostek's sign, Trousseau's sign, tooth decay, rickets, osteoporosis, osteomalacia<br>*Toxicity* (hypercalcemia): Drowsiness, lethargy, muscle flaccidity, nausea, vomiting, constipation, polyuria, polydipsia, pathologic fractures |
| **CHLORIDE** | | |
| Fruits, vegetables, table salt | Maintenance of fluid, electrolyte, acid-base, and osmotic pressure balance | *Deficiency* (rare): Hypochloremic alkalosis<br>*Toxicity:* No known effects |
| **MAGNESIUM*** | | |
| Green leafy vegetables, nuts, seafood, cocoa, whole grains | Acid-base balance, calcium and phosphorus metabolism in bones, muscle relaxation, cellular respiration, nerve impulse transmission, cardiac muscle function and maintenance | *Deficiency* (hypomagnesemia): Confusion, disorientation, easily aroused anger, nervousness, irritability, rapid pulse, tremors, loss of muscle control, neuromuscular dysfunction<br>*Toxicity:* (hypermagnesemia): Drowsiness, lethargy, bradycardia, hypotension, hyporeflexia, nausea |
| **PHOSPHORUS*** | | |
| Eggs, fish, grains, meats, poultry, yellow cheese, milk, milk products | Bone and tooth formation, cell growth and repair, energy production, kidney function, metabolism (carbohydrates, fats, proteins), myocardial contraction, nerve and muscle activity, acid-base balance | *Deficiency* (hypophosphatemia): Appetite loss, fatigue, irregular breathing, nervous disorders, ataxia, paresthesias, muscle weakness<br>*Toxicity* (hyperphosphatemia): tetany, soft-tissue calcification |
| **POTASSIUM** | | |
| Seafood, molasses, bananas, peaches, peanuts, raisins | Heartbeat, muscle contraction, nerve impulse transmission, fluid distribution and osmotic pressure balance, acid-base balance | *Deficiency* (hypokalemia): Dysrhythmias, general muscle weakness, leg cramps, insomnia, nervousness, irritability, anorexia, vomiting, slow, irregular heartbeat, weak reflexes<br>*Toxicity* (hyperkalemia): Bradycardia, apathy, confusion, hyperreflexia progressing to flaccid weakness, oliguria, anuria |

continued

*For specific RDAs, see Appendix A; RDAs for other minerals have not been established.

**MINERALS** continued

| MAIN FOOD SOURCES | MAJOR FUNCTIONS | DEFICIENCY AND TOXICITY FINDINGS |
|---|---|---|
| **SODIUM** | | |
| Seafood, cheese, milk, salt | Extracellular fluid, osmotic pressure balance, muscle contraction, acid-base and water balance, cell permeability, muscle function, nerve impulse transmission | *Deficiency* (hyponatremia): Headache, nausea, vomiting, appetite loss, muscle atrophy, weight loss, hypotension, dry mucous membranes<br>*Toxicity* (hypernatremia): Weight gain, hypertension, thirst, dry mucous membranes, irritability |
| **SULFUR** | | |
| Milk, meats, legumes, eggs | Collagen synthesis, vitamin B formation, muscle metabolism, toxin neutralization, blood clotting | *Deficiency:* No known effects<br>*Toxicity:* No known effects |
| **TRACE ELEMENTS** | | |
| **CHROMIUM** | | |
| Clams, meats, cheese, corn oil, whole grains, brewer's yeast | Carbohydrate and lipid metabolism, serum glucose level maintenance | *Deficiency:* Glucose intolerance (in diabetic patients)<br>*Toxicity:* No known effects |
| **COBALT** | | |
| Beef, eggs, fish, milk products, organ meats, pork | Vitamin $B_{12}$ formation | *Deficiency:* See "Vitamin $B_{12}$ deficiency" in *Vitamins,* pages 47 to 49.<br>Toxicity: No known effects |
| **COPPER** | | |
| Organ meats, raisins, seafood (especially oysters), nuts, molasses | Bone formation; healing processes; hemoglobin, red blood cell, and enzyme formation; mental processes; iron use | *Deficiency:* Diarrhea (in infants), general weakness, impaired respiration, skin sores, bone malformations<br>*Toxicity:* Headache, dizziness, heartburn, weakness, nausea, vomiting, diarrhea, Wilson's disease |
| **FLUORIDE (fluorine)** | | |
| Drinking water | Bone and tooth formation | *Deficiency:* Dental caries<br>*Toxicity* (fluorosis): Tooth enamel mottling and discoloration, increased bone density and calcification |
| **IODINE\*** | | |
| Kelp, salt (iodized), seafood | Regulation of basal metabolic rate, cell metabolism | *Deficiency:* Cold hands and feet, dry hair, irritability, nervousness, obesity<br>*Toxicity:* No known effects |

## MINERALS continued

| MAIN FOOD SOURCES | MAJOR FUNCTIONS | DEFICIENCY AND TOXICITY FINDINGS |
|---|---|---|
| **IRON*** | | |
| Eggs, organ meats, poultry, wheat germ, liver, potatoes, enriched breads and cereals, green vegetables, molasses | Growth (in children), hemoglobin production, stress and disease resistance, cellular respiration, oxygen transport, energy production, regulation of biological and chemical reactions | *Deficiency:* Brittle nails, constipation, respiratory problems, tongue soreness or inflammation, anemia, pallor, weakness, cold sensitivity, fatigue *Toxicity* (hemochromatosis): Abdominal cramps and pain, nausea, vomiting, hemosiderosis |
| **MANGANESE** | | |
| Bananas, egg yolks, green leafy vegetables, liver, soybeans, nuts, whole grains, coffee, tea | Enzyme activation, fat and carbohydrate metabolism, skeletal growth, sex hormone production, vitamin $B_1$ metabolism, vitamin E utilization | *Deficiency:* Ataxia, dizziness, hearing disturbances or loss *Toxicity:* Severe neuromuscular disturbances (similar to parkinsonian effects) |
| **MOLYBDENUM** | | |
| Whole grains, legumes, organ meats | Body metabolism | *Deficiency:* No known effects *Toxicity:* No known effects |
| **SELENIUM** | | |
| Seafood, meats, liver, kidneys | Immune mechanisms, mitochondrial ATP synthesis, cellular protection, fat metabolism | *Deficiency:* No known effects *Toxicity:* No known effects |
| **ZINC*** | | |
| Liver, mushrooms, seafood, soybeans, spinach, meat | Burn and wound healing, carbohydrate digestion, metabolism (carbohydrate, fat, protein), prostate gland function, reproductive organ growth and development, taste and smell | *Deficiency:* Delayed sexual maturity, fatigue, loss of smell and taste, poor appetite, prolonged wound healing, retarded growth, skin disorders *Toxicity:* Vomiting, diarrhea, pancreatitis |

*For specific RDAs, see Appendix A; RDAs for other minerals have not been established.

F.  **Dietary requirements:** See Appendix A for recommended dietary allowances (RDAs) for specific minerals

G.  **Sources:** See *Minerals,* pages 53 to 55, for specific information

H.  **Deficiency and toxicity findings:** See *Minerals,* pages 53 to 55, for specific information

## Points to Remember

The term *minerals* in nutrition usually refers to inorganic ions in their elemental form.

Some minerals—including calcium, phosphorus, magnesium, sodium, potassium, and chloride—are needed by the body in relatively large amounts; trace elements are needed in smaller amounts.

During digestion, minerals are broken down into their ionic form for absorption; unabsorbed minerals are eliminated in either urine or feces.

## Glossary

**Ataxia**—condition characterized by impaired coordination, staggering gait, and postural imbalance; may be seen with manganese deficiency

**Inorganic**—pertaining to or composed of chemical compounds that do not contain carbon as the principal element

**Permeability**—ability to allow penetration; refers to the size of diffusing particles relative to the size of membrane pores

**Tetany**—manifestation of an abnormal serum calcium level characterized by muscle cramps and twitching, convulsions, and sharp flexion of the wrist and ankle joints

# Dietary Guidelines

**Learning Objectives**

After studying this section, the reader should be able to:

• Differentiate between the recommended dietary allowances and the U.S. recommended daily allowances.

• Describe the four basic food groups, including the disadvantages in using them as dietary guidelines.

• Discuss two sets of dietary guidelines recommended by the U.S. government.

• Describe the Inverse Pyramid Food Guide.

• List the current dietary recommendations proposed by the American Cancer Society and the American Heart Association.

## XI. Dietary Guidelines

### A. Introduction

1. Dietary guidelines have been developed by U.S. governmental agencies, nutritionists, and special groups to provide recommendations to promote health
2. Guidelines are to be used for:
   a. Identifying nutrients needed
   b. Recommending types and amounts of food required
   c. Pointing out foods to avoid
3. These guidelines have been developed through years of research on both animals and humans

### B. Recommended dietary allowances (RDAs)

1. General information
   a. RDAs identify adequate daily nutritional needs by specifying amounts of nutrients needed by healthy persons to achieve optimal growth and health
   b. RDAs are recommended for average daily amounts that a person should consume regularly
   c. Diet is considered adequate when ⅔ of the RDAs are provided, poor when less are provided
   d. RDAs reflect current data developed by scientists and nutritionists; they are based on statistical probability and are updated every 5 years
   e. RDAs are published by the U.S. government through the National Research Council and are relevant to those living in the U.S. only (For the Canadian recommended daily allowances, see Appendix B.)
2. Recommendations
   a. Include amounts for calories, protein, fat- and water-soluble vitamins, and minerals
   b. Specify recommended amounts by age and sex, and for pregnant and lactating women
   c. See Appendices A and B for RDAs for Americans and Canadians
3. Advantages
   a. Can be used to assess the nutritional quality of diets
   b. Can be used to evaluate the nutritional adequacy of food supplies available to people
   c. Can be used to estimate standards for public-assistance nutritional programs
4. Disadvantages
   a. Do not include all essential nutrients
   b. Apply to healthy individuals only; requirements are altered with illness
   c. Provide estimates for populations, not individuals
   d. Considered too complex for the general public to use

## C. U.S. recommended daily allowances (U.S. RDAs)

1. General information
   a. Created by the U.S. government in 1968 as a standard to allow for nutritional labeling; originally known as the minimum daily requirements (MDRs)
   b. Are standard guidelines for daily essential nutritional requirements
   c. List amounts that are the highest value recommended for each nutrient for a particular age-group that a person should eat every day to stay healthy
   d. Used as a basis for nutritional labeling; food label states a percentage of U.S. RDAs for each nutrient contained in the product
2. Recommendations: Include percentages of recommended amounts of nutrients (see Appendix C for specific U.S. RDAs)
3. Advantages
   a. Can be used to compare the nutrient values of various foods
   b. Can be used to identify the amount of nutrients contained in foods
   c. Provide a margin of safety higher than that provided by the RDAs for determining adequate nutritional intake
4. Disadvantages
   a. Are not specific for age or sex
   b. Are somewhat inconsistent; certain nutrients are listed in high amounts; others are omitted

## D. Basic food groups

1. General information
   a. Translates RDAs into a simple guide for meeting multiple nutritional needs
   b. Groups broad families of food with similar kinds of nutrients
   c. Recommends servings that vary in size and number according to the nutritional needs of a specific age-group or stage of life
   d. Includes *milk and milk products:* milk, cheese, and ice cream
   e. Includes *meat and meat equivalents:* beef, lamb, pork, poultry, eggs, fish, and shellfish; alternate choices include incomplete proteins, such as dried beans and peas, lentils, and nuts
   f. Includes all types of *fruits and vegetables*
   g. Includes *bread and grains:* whole grain, enriched or restored grains, breads, cooked or ready-to-eat cereals, cornmeal, rolled oats, crackers, flour, grits, pastas, and rice
   h. May include a fifth group proposed by the U.S. Department of Agriculture (USDA)—but not widely accepted—that includes fats and sugars, unenriched or refined cereal products, and alcohol
2. Recommendations: See *Basic food groups,* page 60, for specific recommendations

## BASIC FOOD GROUPS

| FOOD SOURCE | NUTRIENTS SUPPLIED | DAILY SERVINGS NEEDED |
|---|---|---|
| **Milk and milk products group** | | |
| Milk or equivalent serving of cheese, yogurt, ice cream, or ice milk | Complete protein; vitamins (A, D [fortified milk], and B [especially riboflavin, $B_6$, and $B_{12}$]); minerals (calcium, magnesium, phosphorus, zinc) | One serving equals 1 cup Children under age 9: two to three servings Children age 9 to 12: three servings Adolescents: four servings Adults: two servings Pregnant women: three servings Lactating women: four servings |
| **Meat and meat equivalents** | | |
| Meat, fish, eggs, poultry, dry beans, peas, seeds, nuts, peanuts, and peanut butter | Complete protein (except legumes, seeds, and nuts, which must be consumed with other protein foods to supply complete protein); vitamins (B complex, A, E, D); minerals (calcium, iodine, iron, phosphorus, magnesium, zinc); essential fatty acids (in seeds) | One serving consists of 2 to 3 oz meat, 4 tbs peanut butter, 2 eggs, or 1 to 1½ cups cooked beans. Two servings needed daily. |
| **Vegetables and fruits group** | | |
| Citrus fruits, tomatoes, dark green and deep yellow vegetables, unpeeled fruits and vegetables, fruits and vegetables with edible seeds (for example, berries) | Incomplete protein; vitamins (A, C, E, B complex); minerals (iron, calcium, magnesium) | One serving consists of ½ cup cooked or juice, or 1 cup raw. Four servings needed daily. |
| **Breads and grains group** | | |
| Whole grain, enriched and fortified breads, cereals, and pasta | Incomplete protein; vitamins (E and B complex); minerals (iron, phosphorus, magnesium, zinc, calcium) | One serving equals 1 slice of bread or ½ to ¾ oz cooked cereal or pasta. Four servings needed daily. |
| **Fats, sweets, and alcohol group** | | |
| Visible fats and oils (cream, cream cheese, butter, fortified margarine, vegetable oils and shortenings, mayonnaise, salad dressing, fish oils, bacon, bacon grease, fatback); sweets (sugar and foods with high sugar content, such as jams, jellies, honey, candy, soft drinks, and other highly sweetened beverages and toppings); alcoholic beverages (beer, wine, liquor) (*Note:* This food group also includes unenriched breads, pastries, and flour products that have negligible nutritional value.) | Minimal, inlcuding fat-soluble vitamins (in fats and fish oils); vitamin E and polyunsaturated fatty acids (in vegetable oils); calcium and iron (in dark molasses). (*Note:* This food group supplies mostly calories.) | None recommended |

From *Metabolic Problems.* NurseReview series. Springhouse, Pa.: Springhouse Corp., 1988, p.9.

3. Advantages
   a. Provides practical criteria for selection of a nutritionally adequate diet
   b. Allows for maximal nutritional benefit with minimal wasted calories
   c. Supplies an adult with ½ to ⅔ of the required daily energy allowance as well as all the required protein, vitamin A, riboflavin, Vitamin C, calcium, and phosphorus
   d. Allows flexibility in personal food choices
4. Disadvantages
   a. Can include foods from the four groups and still have inadequate intake of some nutrients, such as iron; foods in the same group may contain similar nutrients but will supply these nutrients in different amounts, depending on the specific food chosen, the serving size, and the number of servings
   b. Does not include enough of the foods people regularly eat
   c. Is difficult to use when food mixtures or combinations are used
   d. Is difficult to use to assess and classify new food products
   e. Emphasizes including rather than limiting foods; can encourage overeating
   f. Does not consider the caloric value of foods

## E. Dietary guidelines for Americans
1. General information
   a. Formulated in 1977 by the U.S. Senate Select Committee on Nutrition and Human Needs
   b. Designed to help Americans avoid some nutrition-related problems, such as obesity, heart disease, cancer, GI disorders, and diabetes mellitus
2. Recommendations
   a. Maintain proper weight by controlling caloric intake and increasing exercise
   b. Increase intake of complex carbohydrates and natural sugars from 28% to 48% of total daily caloric intake
   c. Reduce intake of refined sugars from 40% to 10% of total daily caloric intake
   d. Reduce fat intake from 40% to 30% of total daily caloric intake, with 10% of this amount in saturated fats, 10% in unsaturated fats, and 10% in polyunsaturated fats
   e. Reduce cholesterol intake to approximately 300 mg/day
   f. Reduce salt intake to 5g (2 + teaspoonfuls)/day
3. Advantages
   a. Designed to promote good nutrition and health
   b. Offer suggestions on how to achieve optimal health and nutrition
4. Disadvantages
   a. Some researchers believe the recommendations are too restrictive
   b. Have been formulated for the entire population, and are not based on individual evaluation and needs

**F. USDA and Department of Health and Human Services (DHHS) guidelines**
1. General information
   a. Were developed in 1980
   b. Provide general guidelines to promote health through proper diet
   c. Include a recommendation for alcohol intake
2. Recommendations
   a. Eat a wide variety of foods
   b. Maintain desirable weight
   c. Avoid excessive intake of fat, saturated fat, and cholesterol
   d. Maintain an adequate intake of dietary starch and fiber
   e. Avoid excessive intake of sugar
   f. Avoid excessive intake of sodium
   g. Drink alcoholic beverages in moderation only
3. Advantages
   a. Can be used by most individuals
   b. Aimed at promoting health through good nutrition
4. Disadvantages
   a. Provide only general recommendations
   b. Do not specify amounts of intake

**G. Inverse Pyramid Food Guide**
1. General information
   a. Devised by J.A.T. Pennington in 1981
   b. Attempts to limit nutrients that may cause health problems if consumed in excess, makes use of available food supplies, and promotes health
   c. Separates food into four groups with four levels of consumption
   d. The four food groups include vegetables and fruits; grains; vegetable, dairy, and meat sources of protein; and luxury foods, such as desserts, sweets, alcohol, and fats
   e. The four levels of consumption include liberal, moderate, very moderate, and sparse
2. Recommendations (see *Inverse pyramid food guide* for more information)
   a. Vegetables, fruits, and grains should be consumed liberally
   b. Vegetable sources of protein should be consumed in liberal amounts
   c. Skim and low-fat dairy products, lean meat, and poultry should be consumed in moderate amounts
   d. Whole milk dairy products, fatty meats and game, nuts, seeds, and eggs should be consumed in very moderate amounts
   e. Luxury foods should be consumed in sparse amounts
3. Advantages
   a. Attempts to limit intake of certain nutrients
   b. Uses available food supplies
   c. Considers diet in health promotion

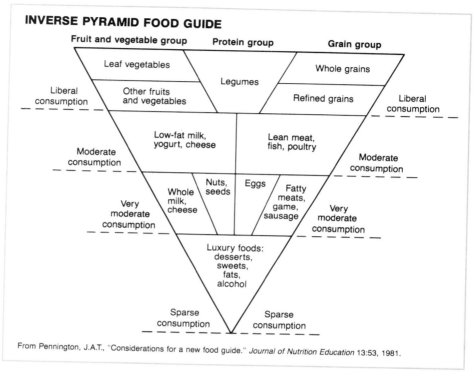

INVERSE PYRAMID FOOD GUIDE

From Pennington, J.A.T., "Considerations for a new food guide." *Journal of Nutrition Education* 13:53, 1981.

4. Disadvantages
   a. Does not specify nutrients
   b. Is somewhat unclear on the distinction among the levels of consumption

## H. American Cancer Society (ACS) guidelines
1. General information
   a. Developed by the ACS in response to recent studies that show that diet may play a major role in cancer prevention
   b. Provide general guidelines for the intake of certain foods shown to increase or decrease the risk of certain types of cancer
2. Recommendations
   a. Avoid obesity
   b. Reduce intake of fats
   c. Increase intake of dietary fiber
   d. Increase daily intake of foods rich in vitamins A and C
   e. Increase intake of cruciferous vegetables, such as cabbage, broccoli, brussels sprouts, kohlrabi, and cauliflower

      f.  Eat salt-cured, smoked, and nitrite-cured foods (such as bacon and certain luncheon meats) in moderation only

      g.  Use alcohol in moderation only

  3.  Advantages: May help a person reduce the risk of developing certain types of cancer

  4.  Disadvantages: Does not provide specific recommended amounts of various nutrients

## I.  American Heart Association (AHA) guidelines

  1.  General information

      a.  Aim to reduce high blood cholesterol levels, one of the major risk factors for developing cardiovascular disease

      b.  Aim to control the amount and types of dietary fat intake and to limit dietary cholesterol intake

  2.  Recommendations for controlling the amount and types of dietary fat intake

      a.  Eat no more than 6 oz of meat, seafood, or poultry daily

      b.  Choose chicken or turkey (without skin) or fish for most meals

      c.  Use lean cuts of meat, trim away all fat before cooking, and discard the fat that cooks out of the meat

      d.  Eat meatless or "low meat" main dishes often

      e.  Limit the use of fats and oils for cooking, baking, and salads to 5 to 8 teaspoonfuls daily

  3.  Recommendations for limiting dietary cholesterol intake

      a.  Eat no more than three egg yolks per week, including those used in cooking or baking

      b.  Limit intake of shrimp, lobster, and organ meats

  4.  Advantages: May help a person reduce the risk of cardiovascular disease

  5.  Disadvantages: May be difficult to maintain compliance

## Points to Remember

Most dietary guidelines consist of general suggestions for diet planning for groups of people rather than specific guidelines for an individual.

Most guidelines are for healthy persons and don't consider the effects of illness on nutritional needs.

All guidelines should be used as a starting point from which to develop a healthy and adequate diet for a particular individual.

## Glossary

**Cruciferous vegetables**—those of the botanical family whose members have cross-like, four-petaled flowers; include cabbage, broccoli, brussels sprouts, kohlrabi, and cauliflower

**Enriched**—nutrients lost in processing have been partially restored

# Nutrition for the Pregnant and Lactating Woman

**Learning Objectives**

After studying this section, the reader should be able to:

• Describe the normal physical and psychosocial characteristics of pregnancy and lactation, as they relate to nutrition.

• List the nutritional requirements during pregnancy and lactation.

• Discuss the nursing implications for promoting healthful nutrition during pregnancy and lactation.

• Discuss the nursing implications for common nutrition-related problems occurring during pregnancy and lactation.

## XII. Nutrition for the Pregnant and Lactating Woman
### A.  Introduction
  1.  A woman's overall nutritional status before conception greatly influences both maternal and infant health
  2.  Relation between maternal prepregnant weight and maternal weight gain during pregnancy is important
      a.  Inadequate maternal weight gain is associated with low-birth-weight (LBW) infants
      b.  Excessive maternal weight gain is associated with increased risk of complications during pregnancy, such as preeclampsia
  3.  Factors affecting maternal nutrition during pregnancy and lactation include age, life-style, cultural and ethnic background, and economic and educational status
  4.  Nutritional needs of all pregnant women depend on the stage of maternal growth and development, prepregnancy maternal nutritional stores, and fetal nutritional demands
  5.  The pregnant adolescent requires additional nutrients to meet two nutritional needs: pregnancy and adolescent growth
  6.  Adolescent pregnancy is considered high-risk because of associated complications, such as preeclampsia and LBW infants
  7.  Advantages of lactation for the woman include:
      a.  Mobilization of fat stores, which helps postpartum weight loss
      b.  Stimulation of uterine contractions by early postpartum feeding, which helps control blood loss and return the uterus to its prepregnant size
      c.  Ready availability of breast milk, which requires no mixing or preparation
      d.  Possible decreased risk of thromboembolism
      e.  Possible decreased risk of breast cancer
      f.  Low cost compared to bottle-feeding
  8.  Disadvantages of lactation for the woman may include:
      a.  Discomfort from breast engorgement and sore or cracked nipples
      b.  Worry about inadequate infant milk intake, because the amount can't be verified
      c.  Reduced milk volume from inadequate caloric intake
  9.  Dietary requirements for non–breast-feeding women return to prepregnancy levels after delivery

### B.  Physical and psychosocial characteristics of pregnancy
  1.  Physical characteristics
      a.  Weight gain during pregnancy typically ranges from 22 to 28 lb (10 to 12.7 kg)
      b.  Metabolic changes include increased basal metabolic rate (BMR), altered glucose tolerance, and impaired folic acid metabolism
      c.  The percentage of total body water increases

      d.  Nausea and vomiting are common during the first trimester
      e.  Appetite and thirst typically increase
      f.  Nausea and heartburn may result from decreased gastric motility and relaxation of the cardiac sphincter
      g.  Hemodilution, possibly leading to physiologic anemia of pregnancy, can result from increased blood volume

  2.  Psychosocial characteristics
      a.  A first pregnancy marks the transition from childlessness to parenthood, a significant developmental milestone
      b.  Pregnancy may be accompanied by stress and anxiety, as manifested in such emotional responses as ambivalence, introversion, and mood swings
      c.  Pregnancy may represent an affirmation of a woman's sexuality by confirming her reproductive ability
      d.  Pregnancy usually requires readjustment of role identity, routines, and family dynamics

**C.  Physical and psychosocial characteristics of a postpartum and lactating woman**
  1.  Physical characteristics
      a.  Weight loss averages approximately 10 to 12 lb (4.5 to 5 kg) immediately after delivery, with additional weight loss occurring over the first few months postpartum
      b.  The uterus gradually returns to its prepregnant size
      c.  Extracellular fluids retained during pregnancy are excreted
      d.  Blood volume returns to prepregnant levels
      e.  Prolactin stimulation promotes milk production in the mammary glands
  2.  Psychosocial characteristics
      a.  The postpartum period represents a time of readjustment and adaptation to major changes in role identity and body image
      b.  This period may be characterized by mood swings and emotional lability, depression, crying, anorexia, and difficulty sleeping resulting from the effects of labor and hormonal changes
      c.  A new mother tends to be passive, somewhat dependent, and preoccupied with her needs during the first day or two after delivery and then begins to act and function independently
      d.  A new mother is more concerned about bodily functions; if breast-feeding, she is concerned about the quantity and quality of her milk and her ability to nurse successfully

**D.  Nutritional requirements**
  1.  General information
      a.  A pregnant woman requires increased levels of all nutrients
      b.  The amount of increase depends on various factors, such as age and prepregnant weight and nutritional status
      c.  Nutritional requirements increase further during lactation

2. Energy (calories)
   a. Pregnancy increases a woman's total daily caloric requirements by an average of 15%. This represents an average increase of 300 calories per day above prepregnant needs, slightly less early in pregnancy and somewhat more later in pregnancy
   b. Factors influencing caloric needs include age, prepregnant weight, height, activity level, and health status
   c. A pregnant adolescent may require more calories than a pregnant adult; up to 50 calories more per day per kg of body weight for a young, growing, physically active adolescent
   d. A lactating woman needs an additional 200 calories per day over her requirements during pregnancy, for an average total intake of 2,500 to 2,700 calories per day
   e. See Appendix A for recommended dietary allowances (RDAs)
3. Protein
   a. Protein requirements increase during pregnancy to provide amino acids for fetal development, blood volume expansion, and growth of maternal tissues
   b. A pregnant adolescent age 11 to 14 requires 1.7 g of protein per kg of body weight per day (g/kg/day); a pregnant adolescent age 15 to 18, 1.5 g/kg/day
   c. Protein requirements increase during lacation because protein is an important ingredient in breast milk
   d. A lactating woman must consume adequate nonprotein calories to prevent the use of protein as an energy source
   d. See Appendix A for RDAs
4. Lipids
   a. Lipids are more completely absorbed during pregnancy; elimination through the bowel is decreased
   b. Requirements vary depending on caloric intake
5. Carbohydrates
   a. Carbohydrates promote maternal weight gain and growth of fetus, placenta, and maternal tissues
   b. Requirements increase during the second and third trimesters
6. Vitamins
   a. Requirements of all fat-soluble vitamins increase during pregnancy and lactation; vitamin K requirements usually can be met through a well-balanced prenatal diet
   b. Serum level of vitamin A decreases slightly in early pregnancy, rises in late pregnancy, then falls before the onset of labor. Pregnant adolescents are prone to vitamin A deficiency
   c. Pregnant adolescents are prone to vitamin D deficiency resulting from inadequate dietary intake

      d. Requirements of all water-soluble vitamins increase during pregnancy and lactation

      e. See Appendix A for RDAs

  7. Minerals

      a. Calcium and phosphorus requirements increase during pregnancy and lactation for energy, cell production, mineralization of fetal bones and teeth, and maintenance of acid-base balance

      b. Absorption and use of calcium is more efficient during pregnancy

      c. Inadequate maternal calcium intake may result in fetal needs being met at the woman's expense

      e. Iodine requirements increase during pregnancy and lactation for fetal thyroid gland development and function

      f. Zinc requirements increase during pregnancy for fetal central nervous system development

      g. Magnesium requirements increase during pregnancy and lactation for fetal cellular metabolism and structural growth

      h. Specific requirements for sodium during pregnancy and lactation have not been established

      i. Iron requirements increase during pregnancy and lactation for fetal red blood cell and hemoglobin production

      j. Because these increased iron requirements cannot be met through dietary intake, iron supplements usually are recommended starting in the second trimester and extending for 2 to 3 months after delivery to replenish depleted maternal iron stores

      k. Pregnant adolescents may have inadequate dietary intake of calcium, phosphorus, zinc, and iron

      l. See Appendix A for RDAs

  8. Fluids

      a. Adequate fluid intake is especially important during lactation; inadequate intake may decrease milk volume

      b. Although no specific fluid requirements have been established, most authorities recommend eight to ten 8-oz glasses per day of water, juice, milk, or soup for a pregnant woman

## E. Promoting healthful nutrition during pregnancy and lactation

  1. General information

      a. Usually, folic acid and iron are the only dietary supplements recommended for pregnant women with adequate diets

      b. Nutritional needs change following delivery, depending on whether the mother breast-feeds

  2. Nursing implications during pregnancy

      a. Assess the pregnant client for nutritional knowledge, cultural and personal dietary preferences, food availability, and dietary needs

      b. Monitor weight gain at least monthly until the 32nd week, then bimonthly until the 36th week, and then weekly until delivery

      c. Explain specific daily dietary requirements

      d. Provide referral to a nutritionist if necessary

  3. Nursing implications for a pregnant adolescent client

      a. Establish a rapport by projecting a relaxed, nonthreatening, nonjudgmental attitude

      b. Provide personalized care and counseling using a positive approach

      c. Assess the home situation carefully

      d. Allow the client to make informed decisions for herself and her baby

      e. Provide concrete information about a nutritionally sound diet, using written and audiovisual materials

      f. Discourage skipping meals and eating inappropriate snack foods

      g. Suggest appropriate nutritious snacks and fast foods

      h. Encourage the client to identify practical ways of improving her diet

      i. Explain the importance of taking nutritional supplements, but also stress that supplements do not decrease the need for a well-balanced diet

      j. Encourage participation in group classes with other pregnant adolescents

  4. Nursing implications during lactation

      a. Explain the specific daily dietary requirements

      b. Instruct in foods that are high in calories, protein, and calcium

      c. Encourage consumption of various fruits and vegetables to provide for the required increases in vitamins and minerals

      d. Encourage the client to drink *at least* eight to ten 8-oz glasses of water daily

      e. Teach the client about manual milk expression and breast-pumping techniques

      f. Teach proper breast and nipple care; encourage the client to wear a support bra

      g. Discuss potential problems, such as inadequate milk flow and breast engorgment, and measures to control or prevent them

      h. Instruct the client to check with her physician before taking any medications because of possible drug transfer to the infant through breast milk

**F. Nursing implications for common nutrition-related problems in pregnancy and lactation**

  1. Lactose intolerance

      a. Observe for the problem especially in Blacks, Mexican-Americans, Native Americans, Ashkenazic Jews, and Orientals

      b. Monitor for difficulty in digesting milk, characterized by such signs and symptoms as abdominal distention, abdominal discomfort or cramps, nausea and vomiting, and loose stools

      c. Explain that tolerance varies among individuals, and that even one glass of milk may produce symptoms in some persons

    d. Advise the client that she may better tolerate milk in cooked form or as cheese and yogurt

    e. Explain that using the enzyme lactose, available in tablet and liquid forms and in lactose-treated milk, may help increase tolerance; instruct the client to check with her physician before using this enzyme

2. Anemia
    a. Monitor hemoglobin level
    b. Assess for pallor and extreme fatigue
    c. Monitor dietary iron intake; point out foods with high iron content
    d. Stress the need for iron supplements; point out such potential adverse effects as nausea and constipation

3. Pica
    a. Be aware that although pica is most commonly practiced in poverty-stricken areas, it occurs in women of all socioeconomic levels; it's often traditional in certain communities or families
    b. Determine the amount consumed of such substances as dirt, clay, starch, and freezer frost
    c. Maintain a nonjudgmental attitude
    d. Discuss the client's feelings about the practice
    e. Provide client teaching aimed at decreasing or eliminating this practice

4. Excessive weight gain
    a. Be aware of normal weight gain: 22 to 28 lb (10 to 12.7 kg) total, broken down into 2 to 4½ lb (1 to 2 kg) in the first trimester and 1 lb (0.4 kg) per week throughout the second and third trimesters
    b. Monitor for excessive or too-rapid weight gain of more than 3 to 5 lb (1.4 to 2.3 kg) per week or more than 6½ lb (3 kg) per month
    c. Assess for fluid retention and overeating
    d. Direct nutritional counseling toward achieving an ideal weight gain of no more than 1 lb per week
    e. Focus on maintaining a caloric intake in accordance with RDA guidelines

5. Inadequate weight gain
    a. Be aware of clients at possible risk for inadequate weight gain: those who are 10% or more below their recommended weight before conception or who have gained less than 22 lb (10 kg) during pregnancy
    b. Assess for factors leading to inadequate weight gain
    c. Advise the client to increase her total daily caloric intake by 500 calories above her prepregnant RDA
    d. Advise the client to increase her daily consumption of protein by 20 g per day
    e. Perform a calorie count to evaluate the client's compliance with these instructions

f.  Set a feasible goal for weight gain; usually a combination of the amount the client is underweight plus 25 lb

6.  Mild preeclampsia

a.  Monitor weight gain and report any too-rapid or excessive increase
b.  Monitor blood pressure and report consistently elevated readings
c.  Assess for edema in the face, hands, and dependent areas such as the ankles
d.  Explain the need for a well-balanced diet
e.  Advise restricting sodium intake to no more than 6 g/day
f.  Monitor for proteinuria; instruct the client to increase protein intake to 80 to 100 g/day to replace protein if excessive amounts are being excreted in urine

## Points to Remember

A woman's overall nutritional status before conception greatly influences both maternal and infant health.

Nutritional requirements increase significantly during pregnancy and lactation.

Inadequate maternal weight gain is associated with LBW infants; excessive maternal weight gain is associated with increased risk of complications of pregnancy, such as preeclampsia.

Adolescent pregnancy is considered high-risk and is associated with an increased risk of such complications as preeclampsia and LBW infants.

## Glossary

**Hemodilution**—increase in the fluid content of blood

**Lactation**—secretion of milk by the mammary glands

**Pica**—Ingestion of nonfood substances, such as dirt or clay

**Preeclampsia**—toxemia of late pregnancy, characterized by hypertension, edema, and proteinuria

**Trimester**—period of approximately 3 months into which the gestation period is divided

# Nutrition for the Infant

**Learning Objectives**

After studying this section, the reader should be able to:

- Describe normal physical and psychosocial characteristics of infancy as they relate to nutrition.

- List nutritional requirements during infancy.

- Discuss nursing implications related to breast-feeding, bottle-feeding, and introducing solid foods to the infant.

- Discuss nursing implications for common nutrition-related problems during infancy.

## XIII. Nutrition for the Infant

### A. Introduction
1. *Infancy* extends from birth to age 12 months; *neonatal* specifically refers to the first 28 days of life
2. Infant feeding practices have changed significantly in the 20th century
3. Nutrients must be supplied to meet the rapid rate of physical growth and development and to promote optimal psychosocial development
4. Development of sound eating habits should begin in infancy
5. Feedings generally decrease from six to eight per day to three to four per day when the infant is between ages 6 and 12 months
6. Acceptable feeding alternatives include human breast milk, commercially prepared cow's milk formula, modified cow's milk formula, and soybean formula

### B. Normal growth and development
1. Physical characteristics
   a. Infancy is a period of rapid growth: weight usually doubles from birth to ages 5 to 6 months and triples by ages 10 to 12 months; length increases by 50% from birth to age 12 months
   b. At birth, the infant has sucking, rooting, and swallowing reflexes; feels hunger and indicates desire for food by crying; and expresses satiety by falling asleep
   c. At age 1 month, the infant has a strong extrusion reflex
   d. At ages 3 to 4 months, the extrusion reflex fades and the infant begins to develop hand-eye coordination
   e. At ages 4 to 5 months, the infant can move the rim of a cup to his lips
   f. At ages 5 to 6 months, the infant can use his fingers to feed himself a cracker
   g. At ages 6 to 7 months, the infant can chew and bite and can hold his own bottle but may not drink from it, preferring that it be held by someone else
   h. At ages 7 to 9 months, the infant demonstrates taste preferences; may refuse food by keeping his lips closed; can hold a spoon and play with it during feeding; can drink from a cup with assistance; and may drink from a straw
   i. At ages 9 to 12 months, the infant can pick up small foods or morsels of food (finger foods) and feed himself; hold his own bottle and drink from it; drink from a cup without assistance but with some spillage; and use a spoon with much spillage
2. Psychosocial characteristics
   a. The infant makes his needs known by crying
   b. The infant develops a sense of trust and attachment
   c. The infant begins a maturation and learning process, demonstrating specific behaviors regarding food

## C. Nutritional requirements

1. General information
   a. Nutritional requirements during infancy generally are based on the average level of energy and nutrients contained in human milk (with the exception of fluoride, vitamin D, and iron)
   b. High levels of nutrients and calories are required to support growth and development
   c. Nutritional requirements change as the infant grows and develops
   d. Dietary supplements may be required in cases of a nutrient-deficient diet
2. Energy (calories)
   a. Caloric requirements decrease gradually from birth to age 1
   b. See Appendix A for recommended dietary allowances (RDAs)
3. Protein
   a. Protein requirements are highest during the first 6 months of life
   b. Requirements are adjusted to reflect the infant's size and rate of growth
   c. See Appendix A for RDAs
4. Lipids
   a. Dietary fats must be readily digestible and absorbable by the infant
   b. Fats should comprise 30% to 50% of an infant's total daily caloric intake
   c. Approximately 3% of the total caloric intake should be in the form of linoleic acid, an essential fatty acid
   d. Human milk and cow's milk provide 48% to 54% of their calories as fat; commercial infant formulas, 36% to 38%
5. Carbohydrates should comprise 30% to 60% of an infant's total daily caloric intake
6. Vitamins and minerals
   a. Infants require the same vitamins and minerals as adults, but in different amounts
   b. An infant's vitamin and mineral requirements are influenced by the amount of nutrients received and stored in utero, the growth rate, and the caloric and protein intake
   c. Commercial infant formulas are fortified with selected vitamins and minerals
   d. An infant with depleted or inadequate iron stores may require dietary iron supplements
   e. See Appendix A for RDAs
7. Fluids
   a. Infants have a greater need for water than do adults
   b. Infants have a larger percentage of body weight in water (70% to 75%) than do adults (60% to 65%)
   c. An infant's kidneys are unable to concentrate urine and conserve water efficiently
   d. An infant obtains dietary water predominantly from breast milk or commercial infant formula

e.  Water requirements increase in warm weather or during periods of elevated body temperature
f.  RDA at birth: approximately 150 ml/kg of body weight/day
g.  RDA at age 3 months: 140 to 160 ml/kg/day; range of 750 to 850 ml/day
h.  RDA at age 6 months: 130 to 135 ml/kg/day; range of 950 to 1,100 ml/day
i.  RDA at age 9 months: 125 to 145 ml/kg/day; range of 1,100 to 1,250 ml/day
j.  RDA at age 1 year: 120 to 135 ml/kg/day; range of 1,150 to 1,300 ml/day

## D.  Breast-feeding

1.  General information
    a.  Breast-feeding is the preferred form of nutrition recommended by the American Academy of Pediatrics for full-term infants
    b.  Three types of breast milk are produced during lactation: *colostrum, transitional milk,* and *mature milk*
    c.  *Colostrum* is a yellowish or creamy-appearing fluid; contains more protein, fat-soluble vitamins, and minerals than mature breast milk and high levels of immunoglobulins
    d.  *Transitional milk* replaces colostrum within 2 to 4 days after delivery; it contains higher levels of fat, lactose, water-soluble vitamins, and calories than colostrum
    e.  *Mature milk* is the final milk produced, usually by the third or fourth day after delivery; it contains a high percentage of water and provides 20 calories per oz
    f.  Maternal factors leading to the success of breast-feeding include attitudes and expectations toward breast-feeding; woman's desire to breast-feed; knowledge about milk production and breast-feeding practices; availability of support systems; appropriate life-style and career; and adequate nutritional status and dietary intake

2.  Advantages of breast-feeding
    a.  Breast-feeding is the most economical form of feeding; however, it isn't "free" milk, because a lactating woman needs a high-protein, high-carbohydrate diet
    b.  Breast milk is readily available at all times
    c.  Breast milk is naturally free of contamination and eliminates the need to sterilize bottles and nipples
    d.  Breast milk provides immunologic benefits to the infant
    e.  Breast-feeding greatly reduces the risk of overfeeding
    f.  Breast-feeding promotes a close maternal-child relationship

3.  Disadvantages of breast-feeding
    a.  Breast-feeding may cause a woman to feel a loss of freedom and independence

b. Most drugs taken by the woman who is breast-feeding an infant are transmitted through the breast milk to the nursing infant
c. An inadequate caloric intake can reduce milk volume, although milk quality remains unaffected
4. Nursing implications: Teach the breast-feeding woman to
a. Use rooming-in
b. Encourage frequent and early breast-feeding following delivery
c. Manually express milk and use correct technique for pumping breasts
d. Select among various breast-feeding positions and alternate breasts at each feeding
e. Recognize normal feeding behaviors of an infant
f. Burp and position the infant after feeding
g. Investigate breast-feeding support groups, such as the La Leche League
h. When appropriate, wean her infant from breast milk

**E. Bottle-feeding**
1. General information
a. Bottle-feeding may use various commercially prepared milk- or soy-based formulas
b. These formulas contain mostly saturated fatty acids, differing amounts of amino acids, and higher protein, calcium, sodium and chloride levels than breast milk
2. Advantages of bottle-feeding
a. Bottle-feeding provides a suitable alternative to breast-feeding
b. Bottle-feeding is less restrictive to the woman than breast-feeding
c. Bottle-feeding allows a more accurate assessment of the infant's intake than does breast-feeding
d. Bottle-feeding may be indicated for an infant with a congenital anomaly, such as cleft palate, that interferes with breast-feeding
e. Bottle-feeding may be necessary if an infant requires a special formula as a result of allergies or inborn errors of metabolism
3. Disadvantages of bottle-feeding
a. Bottle formulas may be more difficult for the infant to digest than breast milk
b. Bottle formulas are more expensive, and more time-consuming to prepare than breast milk; mistakes may be made in mixing formulas
4. Nursing implications: Teach the mother of a bottle-feeding infant to
a. Investigate the various types of formulas available (ready-to-use, concentrated liquid, powder) and their preparation methods
b. Make sure the hole in the nipple is large enough for milk to drip out when the bottle is held still
c. Hold the infant in a position similar to that used for breast-feeding
d. Hold the infant during feeding; do not prop the bottle

     e. Point the nipple directly into the infant's mouth, not toward the palate or tongue, and place it on top of the tongue; keep the nipple full of formula to minimize air swallowing

     f. Feed the infant usually every 4 hours, or about six times a day

     g. Make sure the infant retains about 2 to 3 oz of formula at each feeding

     h. Hold the infant upright against the shoulder for burping

     i. Burp the infant at regular intervals, preferably at the middle and end of the feeding or after each ounce of formula is ingested

     j. Discourage overfeeding; do not force the infant to finish the bottle

     k. Discourage unscheduled feeding as a response to crying

**F. Solid foods**

  1. General information

     a. Usually, solid foods may be added to an infant's diet by ages 5 to 6 months

     b. Introducing solid foods should not be delayed beyond ages 7 to 9 months

     c. An infant's first solid foods should be strained, pureed, or mashed

     d. The amount of solid food at each meal should progress from 1 to 2 teaspoonfuls initially to ¼ to ½ cup as the infant grows

     e. An infant usually can start eating "finger foods" by ages 6 to 7 months

     f. An infant usually can start eating chopped table food or commercially prepared junior food by ages 9 to 12 months

     g. The order in which solid foods are added to an infant's diet can vary; however, most authorities recommend the following order: cereals (rice cereal is usually started first because it has a low risk for allergic reaction), vegetables, fruits, meats

     i. A breast-fed infant requires more high-protein foods than does a formula-fed infant

  2. Nursing implications: Teach the mother to

     a. Mix cereal with breast milk, formula, or water

     b. Discontinue—with the physician's approval—iron supplements once cereal has been introduced to the infant's diet

     c. Offer new foods one at a time and early in the feeding session while the infant is still hungry

     d. Start the infant with fruits that are generally well-tolerated, such as applesauce, bananas, and pears

     e. Avoid prepared fruits and vegetables not specifically designed for infants

     f. Offer fruit juice only from a cup, not a bottle

     g. Avoid fatty meats

     h. Prepare meat, fish, and poultry by baking, broiling, steaming, or poaching

     i. Include organ meats

     j. Make sure that soup contains only foods that have been introduced into the diet

k. Serve egg yolk hard-boiled and mashed, soft-boiled, or poached
l. Introduce egg white in small quantities (1 teaspoonful) toward the end of the first year to detect any allergic reactions
m. Use cheese as a substitute for meat and as a "finger food"
n. Supervise all meals and snacks
o. Be sure that food can be chewed easily by the infant
p. Be aware that candy, nuts, grapes, hot dogs, raw carrots, tough meats, and popcorn are associated with choking
q. Remember that the infant should not eat or drink from a cup while lying down, playing, or strapped in a car seat
r. Cook foods until tender
s. Serve food in small pieces
t. Be aware that topical teething anesthetics can interfere with the infant's ability to swallow foods that must be chewed thoroughly

## G. Nursing implications for common nutrition-related problems

1. Regurgitation or vomiting
   a. Assess the infant for possible GI abnormalities
   b. Encourage the mother to feed the infant slowly and to pause several times during the feeding
   c. Instruct the mother to burp the infant often during feeding
   d. Instruct the mother to hold the infant in an upright position during feeding
   e. Teach the mother to place the infant on his stomach or side after feeding to prevent aspiration
   f. Tell the mother to notify the physician if regurgitation or vomiting persists
2. Constipation
   a. Assess the amount and frequency of milk and water feedings; if necessary, suggest that the mother give the infant water between regular feedings
   b. With the physician's approval, encourage the mother to increase the amount or frequency of feedings, or both, and to add high-fiber foods to the infant's diet
   c. Encourage the mother to provide a quiet, relaxed atmosphere during feedings
   d. Instruct the mother to notify the physician if infant constipation persists
3. Diarrhea
   a. Assess the amount and character of the infant's stools
   b. Assess the infant's skin turgor as an indicator of his hydration status
   c. Evaluate the infant's feeding patterns and suggest changes as necessary
   d. Instruct the mother to notify the physician if diarrhea persists

4. Hiccups
   a. Encourage the mother to offer the infant water between feedings
   b. Instruct the mother to burp the infant often during feedings
   c. Encourage the mother to provide a quiet, relaxed atmosphere during feedings
5. Colic
   a. Encourage the mother to provide a quiet, relaxed atmosphere during feedings
   b. Tell the mother to feed the infant slowly and to pause several times during the feeding
   c. Instruct the mother to burp the infant often during feeding
   d. Teach the mother measures to promote infant comfort, such as stroking, caressing, and rocking

## Points to Remember

Infancy is a period of rapid growth; nutritional and caloric requirements are high.

The infant's eating habits grow increasingly sophisticated, which changes the type of foods he is able to ingest.

The selection of a feeding method for the neonate—either breast-feeding or bottle-feeding—is one of the mother's major decisions with significant nutritional, economic, and psychological implications.

Sound eating habits must begin in infancy.

## Glossary

**Colostrum**—thin, yellowish, milky fluid secreted by the mammary glands during pregnancy and in the first several days postpartum

**Extrusion reflex**—normal reflex response in infants; when the infant's tongue is touched or depressed, he pushes the tongue outward

**La Leche League**—organization that provides education, support, and assistance to breast-feeding women

**Rooting reflex**—normal reflex response in infants; when the infant's mouth is touched or stroked, he turns his head toward the stimulated side and begins to suck

**Weaning**—process of discontinuing breast-feeding or bottle-feeding while beginning another feeding method

# Nutrition for the Toddler and Preschool-Age Child

**Learning Objectives**

After studying this section, the reader should be able to:

• Describe the normal physical and psychosocial characteristics of early childhood as they relate to nutrition.

• List the nutritional requirements during early childhood.

• Discuss the nursing implications for promoting healthful nutrition during early childhood.

• Discuss important nursing implications for common nutrition-related problems in early childhood.

## XIV. Nutrition for the Toddler and Preschool-Age Child

A. **Introduction**
1. *Toddler* refers to a child in the transition period between infancy and preschool, ages 1 to 3
2. *Preschooler* refers to a child ages 3 to 6
3. A toddler requires less food and is not as hungry as an infant; this age is the best time to introduce a child to good food habits
4. Toddlers and preschoolers have basically the same nutritional requirements

B. **Normal growth and development**
1. Physical characteristics
   a. A toddler's growth rate slows from ages 1 to 1½, with weight increasing about 5 to 10 lb (2.5 kg to 5 kg); birth weight typically quadruples by age 2½, with increased muscle mass accounting for about half of the total weight gain; growth rate is approximately 3″ (7.5 cm) per year from ages 1 to 3; overall rate of skeletal growth slows
   b. A child achieves many important developmental milestones associated with feeding. By ages 1 to 1½, a toddler usually drools less, can drink well from a cup but may drop it when finished, and holds a cup with both hands. By age 2, he can use a straw, chew food with the mouth closed, shift food in the mouth (which aids chemical digestion), distinguish between "finger foods" and foods eaten with utensils, and hold a small glass in one hand. By age 3, the toddler can use a spoon with little spillage and begin to use a fork properly, and uses an adult chewing pattern, which involves a rotary jaw action
   c. During the preschool period, growth continues at a slow, uneven rate. Weight increases about 3 to 5 lb (1.5 to 2.5 kg) per year; height, about 2½″ (6.4 cm) per year. Bones and muscles grow larger and stronger. Because of a proportionately greater increase in height relative to weight, the chubby appearance of a toddler will probably give way to a leaner body shape
   d. Fine motor movements continue to develop in the preschool period, with an increase in dexterity in handling eating utensils. By age 4, the child rarely spills food from a spoon, serves himself finger foods, and eats with a fork held properly in the fingers. By age 4½, the child uses a fork instead of a spoon when appropriate
2. Psychosocial characteristics
   a. During the toddler period, a child typically strives for a sense of self-control through such behaviors as demanding to feed himself, refusing to eat, and requesting or refusing certain foods
   b. The toddler also may have a short attention span and be easily distracted, making it difficult for him to sit still for meals
   c. The toddler may exhibit ritualism related to eating, such as insisting on using a special cup or bowl; such behavior provides a sense of security

 d. As the toddler gradually grows less self-centered and directs more attention to the outside world, his mouth and hands become important means of gaining information. He may be a messy eater, unable at times to differentiate between edible and inedible items
 e. In the preschool period, a child begins to interpret information about food from parents and other people around him and incorporate it into his value system about food
 f. The preschooler is bombarded with food messages from television; his limited experience makes it difficult for him to evaluate this information accurately
 g. The preschooler begins to associate certain foods with social occasions and behaviors. If food is used inappropriately to reward, punish, or bribe a child, eating may have unpleasant connotations
 h. The preschooler enjoys imitating adult behavior and acting out real-life situations, such as grocery shopping and preparing and serving meals. During this period, he begins to integrate the food habits he observes in adults—both good and bad habits—into his own behavior
 i. Sibling relationships become increasingly important as the child grows. A preschooler typically emulates an older brother or sister, including food habits
 j. A preschooler's eating behaviors may change during periods of stress, such as the arrival of a new baby at home, illness, moving, or breakup of the family
 k. Many preschoolers are enrolled in nursery or day-care programs that include meals or snacks as part of the daily activities. In such programs, the kind of food and manner in which it is presented have a significant impact on the child. Ideally, he learns that mealtime is an opportunity for socializing and sharing with others

## C. Nutritional requirements
 1. General information
   a. Compared to infants, toddlers and preschoolers usually have high activity levels but slowed growth rates, resulting in increased requirements for some nutrients and decreased requirements for others
   b. Poor nutritional status in toddlers and preschoolers is most common in lower socioeconomic groups, where the amount and variety of available foods may be limited
 2. Energy (calories)
   a. A toddler's daily caloric requirements are less than an infant's
   b. A preschooler has basically the same caloric requirements as a toddler
   c. See Appendix A for recommended dietary allowances (RDAs)
 3. Protein
   a. A toddler's daily protein requirements are slightly lower than an infant's
   b. A preschooler has basically the same protein requirements as a toddler
   c. See Appendix A for RDAs

4. Lipids. A toddler and a preschooler both require about 30% to 50% of their daily caloric intake as fats
5. Carbohydrates
   a. No specific age-related requirements have been established
   b. Most authorities recommend that 50% to 60% of the total daily caloric intake be supplied as carbohydrates
6. Vitamins
   a. Vitamin requirements for toddlers and preschoolers are slightly greater than those for an infant
   b. An adequate vitamin D level is especially important for proper skeletal growth and calcium metabolism. A child's daily vitamin D requirements depend on his geographic location and amount of sunlight exposure
   c. See Appendix A for RDAs
7. Minerals
   a. A toddler's mineral requirements are slightly greater than an infant's. Adequate calcium and phosphorus are needed for bone mineralization
   b. A toddler's daily iron, calcium, and phosphorus requirements may be difficult to meet because of his characteristically poor eating habits
   c. A preschooler's mineral requirements remain high as growth and development progress. A varied diet usually provides adequate amounts of each mineral
   d. Calcium requirements remain steady throughout these two age-groups
   e. See Appendix A for RDAs
8. Fluids
   a. A toddler requires approximately 115 ml/kg of fluid daily, reduced fluid requirement from infancy because growth decreases total body water
   b. A preschooler requires slightly more than 100 ml/kg of fluid daily; exact requirements depend on activity level, climate, and health status

**D. Promoting healthful nutrition in early childhood**
1. General information
   a. The eating habits a child forms during the toddler and preschool years provide the basis for future nutritional patterns
   b. More than at any other age, a toddler's or a preschooler's physical and psychosocial development influence dietary habits
   c. Teaching is aimed at both the child and the family
2. Nursing implications: Teach the parents of a toddler to
   a. Allow ample time after play for the child to settle down before eating
   b. Establish a mealtime routine and follow it consistently
   c. Keep distractions to a minimum during mealtimes
   d. Closely supervise the child to prevent ingestion of harmful substances
   e. Make mealtimes enjoyable and stress-free; do not force the child to eat
   f. Provide the child with advance food choices when appropriate
   h. Provide nutritious food in small portions
   i. Serve fewer spicy and more bland foods

       j. Provide favorite, child-sized eating utensils
       k. Provide "finger foods"
       l. Provide foods that are separate; a toddler rarely enjoys such mixed foods as stews or casseroles
   3. Nursing implications: Teach the parents of a preschooler to
       a. Limit the child's intake of nonnutritious foods by not keeping such foods in the home
       b. Maintain a warm, relaxed, and friendly atmosphere at mealtimes
       c. Provide the child with a comfortable chair and appropriately sized utensils and dishes
       d. Establish reasonable rules of behavior for mealtimes, and reinforce desired behavior
       e. Provide an ample variety of foods
       f. Gradually introduce the child to new foods, preferably at the beginning of meals
       g. Cut food into bite-size pieces
       h. Serve food at room temperature if the child prefers
       i. Allow the child to decide when he has had enough to eat

## E. Nursing implications for common nutrition-related problems
   1. Physiological anorexia
       a. Observe for a decrease in the child's food intake at about age 18 months
       b. Encourage the parents to provide various foods, because the child may become a picky eater with strong taste preferences
       c. Explain to the parents that the child may eat a lot one day and almost nothing the next day
       d. Teach the parents about the possible physical and psychosocial changes that may occur and their impact on dietary habits
   2. Nursing-bottle mouth syndrome
       a. Observe for this syndrome in children ages 18 months to 4 years with extensive dental caries and discolored teeth who have a history of prolonged bottle feeding, continuous use of bottles during the daytime, or sleeping with a bottle
       b. Encourage the parents to limit the use of bottles, particularly at bedtime and for dispensing fruit juices
   3. Decreased food intake in a preschooler
       a. Explain to the parents that a preschooler usually doesn't need as much food as a toddler, and that his appetite will vary depending on his growth rate and activity level
       b. Observe for such signs and symptoms as fatigue, emotional stress associated with mealtime, attention-seeking behavior, dental caries or mouth pain, and any psychological disturbance or physical illness that can cause a reduction in food intake
   4. Manipulative behavior
       a. Explain to the parents that toddlers and preschoolers often attempt to manipulate their parents by modifying their eating habits in ways they know the parents will find troublesome

    b. Teach the parents that coaxing or forcing the toddler or preschooler to eat may further increase the manipulative behavior

    c. Explain to the parents that the child may use manipulative behavior as he discovers the nonnutritional function of food; for example, when parents use food as a reward or withhold it as a punishment

5. Food jags

    a. Explain to the parents that food jags usually are transient and represent no cause for alarm

    b. Tell the parents to continue offering the child variety without making an issue of his behavior

6. Pica

    a. Observe the child for ingestion of nonfood substances; some children with pica are deficient in iron

    b. Particularly observe for this behavior in children of lower socioeconomic backgrounds

7. Lead poisoning

    a. Be aware of lead poisoning's serious effects on the nervous system, kidneys, and bone marrow

    b. Be aware that lead absorption decreases with the regular consumption of a well-balanced diet

    c. Assess the child for changes in neurologic status

    d. Instruct the parents to remove all lead-based paint from the home in accordance with accepted safety standards

## Points to Remember

The period from birth until the child enters school is the time of greatest parental influence on the formation of the child's nutritional patterns.

The eating habits that a toddler learns may have lasting effects on his nutritional status.

Nutritional requirements for preschoolers are fairly similar to those for toddlers.

## Glossary

**Caries**—tooth decay

**Food jags**—changes in the child's established eating pattern, such as refusing to eat a food previously enjoyed or eating only one food for several days; common behavior in a preschool child

**Physiologic anorexia**—phenomenon often manifested in toddlers in which they become picky eaters with strong taste preferences

# Nutrition for the School-Age Child

**Learning Objectives**

After studying this section, the reader should be able to:

• Describe the normal physical and psychosocial characteristics of school-age children as they relate to nutrition.

• List the nutritional requirements for school-age children.

• Discuss the nursing implications for promoting healthful nutrition during the school-age years.

• Discuss the nursing implications for common nutrition-related problems affecting school-age children.

## XV. Nutrition for the School-Age Child

A. **Introduction**
   1. *School age* refers to the period from ages 6 to 12
   2. During this period, often called the latent-growth period, growth rate slows and body changes occur gradually
   3. Reserves for the rapid growth in adolescence are being developed
   4. By the latter part of this period, girls usually experience a faster rate of growth and development than boys

B. **Normal growth and development**
   1. Physical characteristics
      a. Growth proceeds at a slow pace, marked by small spurts and plateaus. Weight increases an average of 7 lb (3.2 kg) per year; height, an average of 2½" (6.4 cm) per year
      b. Weight and height vary greatly
      c. Deciduous teeth are shed and replaced by permanent teeth
      d. The school-age child also reaches several important developmental milestones associated with feeding. By age 6, the child can spread food with a knife. By age 7, the child can cut food with a knife
   2. Psychosocial characteristics
      a. During the school-age years, a child develops a sense of industry and pride in accomplishment
      b. The child spends increasing amounts of time away from home with friends and at school and is subject to increased influence of school friends and adults other than his parents on his food habits. He may emphatically reject food his parents try to force him to eat
      c. Stress related to schoolwork, outside activities, or illness may influence the child's appetite; for instance, a child involved in outside activities may be reluctant to stop and eat

C. **Nutritional requirements**
   1. General information
      a. Growth remains slow and steady; the body continues to stockpile reserves for adolescence
      b. A school-age child's nutritional requirements are similar to or slightly greater than a preschooler's
   2. Energy (calories)
      a. The recommended daily caloric intake for a school-age child is 86 calories/kg of body weight/day
      b. See Appendix A for recommended dietary allowances (RDAs)
   3. Protein
      a. Most authorities recommend that 10% to 15% of a school-age child's total daily caloric intake be supplied as protein
      b. See Appendix A for RDAs

4.  Lipids
    a.  No specific age-related requirements have been established
    b.  Most authorities recommend that 25% to 35% of a school-age child's total daily caloric intake be supplied as fats
5.  Carbohydrates
    a.  No specific age-related requirements have been established
    b.  Most authorities recommend that 50% to 60% of a school-age child's total daily caloric intake be supplied as carbohydrates
6.  Vitamins
    a.  Vitamin requirements for school-age children are the same or slightly higher than those for preschoolers
    b.  See Appendix A for RDAs
7.  Minerals
    a.  Calcium requirements remain steady from ages 1 through 10
    b.  Iron and zinc requirements for a school-age child are the same as those for a preschooler
    c.  See Appendix A for RDAs
8.  Fluids
    a.  No specific RDAs for fluid intake have been established
    b.  Most authorities recommend that a school-age child consume about 100 ml of fluid/kg of body weight/day, with the optimum level depending on activity level, climate, and health status

**D.  Promoting healthful nutrition in the school-age child**
1.  General information
    a.  Changes occur gradually during the school-age years
    b.  Children in this age-group continue to form values regarding food
2.  Nursing implications: Teach the parents to
    a.  Reinforce food values
    b.  Continue to emphasize and reinforce appropriate food practices
    c.  Teach the child how to evaluate information about food and nutrition
    d.  Introduce the idea that the media, including television, do not always provide the most reliable information about nutrition
    e.  Monitor whether school lunches provide needed nutrients
    f.  Provide carefully planned, nutritionally balanced bag lunches
    g.  Provide nutritious snacks as supplements to regular meals
    h.  Encourage the child to make sound nutritional choices when he chooses his own food away from home

**E.  Nursing implications for common nutrition-related problems**
1.  Skipping breakfast
    a.  Encourage parents to teach the child how to prepare his own simple breakfast
    b.  Instruct parents to provide breakfast foods that the child likes

    c. Encourage parents to enroll the child in a school breakfast program if one is available and the child is eligible

2. Obesity
    a. Work with the child to modify his eating habits, incorporating good habits and eliminating bad ones
    b. Have parents monitor the amount of time the child spends in sedentary activities, such as watching television, and encourage him to increase his activity level
    c. Observe the child during stressful times to see if he eats more as a way of dealing with stress

## Points to Remember

Resources for the increased growth needs of the adolescent period are being developed during the school-age years.

Upon entering school, the child develops an eating style that is increasingly independent of parental influence.

Nutritional education should continue throughout the school-age years as part of the child's enlarging knowledge.

## Glossary

**Deciduous teeth**—refers to the 20 teeth appearing during infancy, consisting of 4 incisors, 2 canines, and 4 molars in each jaw; replaced by permanent teeth

**Industry**—developmental task of the school-age child demonstrated by a desire to engage in tasks and achieve success in all activities

**Latent**—present with the potential for becoming active, but now hidden or undeveloped; refers to the growth period of the school-age child characterized by a slow growth rate and gradual body changes

**Sedentary**—characterized by physical inactivity

# Nutrition for the Adolescent

## Learning Objectives

After studying this section, the reader should be able to:

• Describe the normal physical and psychosocial characteristics of adolescence as they relate to nutrition.

• List the nutritional requirements for adolescents.

• Discuss the nursing implications for promoting healthful nutrition during adolescence.

• Discuss the nursing implications for common nutrition-related problems affecting adolescents.

## XVI. Nutrition for the Adolescent

### A. Introduction

1. *Adolescence* refers to the transitional stage linking childhood to adulthood, extending from ages 10 to 18
2. Adolescence is a period of rapid physical, emotional, social, and sexual change
3. Limited reliable data are available regarding growth, development, and nutritional needs during adolescence; data suggest that nutritional requirements peak during adolescence
4. Nutritional problems from childhood may intensify during adolescence because of increased physical needs and growth

### B. Normal growth and development

1. Physical characteristics
   a. Growth rate increases during early adolescence, but rates differ between girls and boys. In girls, the growth spurt begins between ages 10 and 12, peaks at age 12, and is completed by age 15. In boys, the growth spurt begins between ages 12 and 13, peaks at age 14, and is completed by age 19
   b. During adolescence, a boy's weight typically doubles, gaining an average of 66 lb (30 kg); girls gain on the average of 49 lb (22 kg)
   c. Body composition also changes. Girls develop a layer of adipose tissue; boys experience a substantial increase in lean body mass
   d. Both sexes achieve sexual maturity; menstruation begins in girls
   e. Growth rate may correlate with sexual maturation; for example, the onset of menses in girls often correlates with the time of greatest growth
2. Psychosocial characteristics
   a. A child in early adolescence behaves much like an older school-age child in being likely to agree with parental suggestions concerning eating habits
   b. In contrast, an older adolescent is struggling to become an adult
   c. A major task for the adolescent is achieving a sense of identity. This involves learning about who he is as a person, what he values, and the direction he will take in adulthood
   d. An adolescent must separate from his parents and family. To do so, he tries out different roles or ways of behaving, which may be reflected in his food habits
   e. The values and opinions of the adolescent's peer group typically exert great influence on his food choices
   f. An adolescent may not relate nutrition to bodily function, but to immediate gratification of a need like hunger
   g. With adequate nutrition, the adolescent may have positive feelings about his body and its changes and capabilities; with inadequate nutrition, he may have poor body performance and develop low self-esteem

## C. Nutritional requirements

1. General information
   a. Requirements for specific nutrients are based on physiologic age rather than on chronologic age
   b. The most common nutritional deficiencies affecting adolescents include iron, calcium, riboflavin, and vitamin A
2. Energy (calories)
   a. More calories are required to maintain lean body tissue than to maintain fat tissue; male adolescents require approximately 500 to 600 more calories per day than female adolescents
   b. See Appendix A for recommended dietary allowances (RDAs)
3. Protein
   a. Most authorities recommend that 7% to 8% of an adolescent's total caloric intake be supplied as protein
   b. Individual protein requirements depend on factors such as sex, age, nutritional status, and protein quality
   c. See Appendix A for RDAs
4. Lipids
   a. No specific age-related requirements have been established
   b. Required levels vary depending on an individual's caloric needs
5. Carbohydrates
   a. No specific age-related requirements have been established
   b. Required levels vary depending on an individual's caloric needs
6. Vitamins
   a. An adolescent has an increased need for thiamin, riboflavin, and niacin because of high energy requirements, and an increased need for vitamin D because of rapid skeletal growth
   b. An adolescent's requirements for vitamins A, C, E, and $B_6$ and folic acid are essentially the same as an adult's
   c. See Appendix A for RDAs
7. Minerals
   a. An adolescent has an increased need for iron to support the increases in lean body mass, blood volume, and hemoglobin level
   b. In females, onset of menstruation increases the need for iron
   c. Zinc requirements increase during growth spurts
   d. Calcium requirements closely parallel the increase in lean body mass and mineral deposits in growing bones. Males require more calcium than females because of their larger skeletal mass
   e. See Appendix A for RDAs
8. Fluids
   a. At age 14, fluid requirements average 50 to 60 ml/kg of body weight/day, for a range between 2,200 and 2,700 ml/day
   b. At age 18, fluid requirements average 40 to 50 ml/kg of body weight/day, for a range between 2,200 and 2,700 ml/day
   c. Required amounts increase with high physical activity level

### D. Promoting healthful nutrition in adolescents

1. General information
   a. Adolescence is a time of great psychosocial development and adjustment
   b. The struggle to leave childhood and enter adulthood may affect an adolescent's food choices and, therefore, nutritional status
2. Nursing implications: Teach parents to
   a. Encourage the adolescent to express his feelings regarding food and eating
   b. Set good nutrition examples
   c. Provide the adolescent with up-to-date information on good nutrition
   d. Encourage the adolescent to become involved in meal planning and food preparation at home
   e. Keep nourishing ready-to-eat foods on hand
   f. Encourage the adolescent to become involved in physical activity for his overall health
   g. Encourage the adolescent to exercise self-direction and take responsibility for his food choices

### E. Nursing implications for common nutrition-related problems

1. Skipping meals and excessive snacking
   a. Teach the adolescent the basic concepts of healthful nutrition, including the components of a well-balanced diet
   b. Teach the adolescent about nutritious snack choices, and encourage him to avoid "junk" foods high in fat, salt, or sugar
   c. Encourage parents to keep nutritious snacks available in the home
   d. Encourage family discussions on nutrition and food habits
   e. Suggest that parents try to set positive examples by demonstrating sound eating habits themselves
   f. Discourage parents from criticizing the adolescent's eating habits; remind them that constructive suggestions work better than criticism
   g. Advise parents to include the adolescent in meal planning and food preparation
2. Obesity
   a. Be aware that an adolescent usually is sensitive about his appearance; avoid criticism
   b. Be aware that obesity may be the focus of family conflict, but not the cause; refer the family to counseling, as necessary
   c. Help the adolescent set realistic goals for weight loss
   d. Teach the adolescent how to balance intake of calories to ensure normal growth while still losing weight
   e. Encourage involvement in the small-group approach to weight problems, such as Weight Watchers
   f. Focus group activities on peer support and physical activities

3. Cigarettes, alcohol, drugs
   a. Teach the adolescent the damaging effects of cigarettes, alcohol, and drugs on nutrients, nutritional status, and physical health and well-being
   b. Be alert to changes in eating habits that may signal possible substance abuse problems
   c. Offer support and guidance; encourage involvement of peers in discussing potential problems and hazards
   d. Refer the adolescent for counseling, as necessary
4. Acne vulgaris
   a. Explain that, according to available evidence, diet has no major role in causing acne; eliminating such foods as chocolate, nuts, fried and fatty food, and soft drinks has no proven effect on controlling acne
   b. Be aware that the adolescent will be extremely self-conscious when his face has "broken out"
   c. Offer guidance and support; encourage scrupulous hygiene and use of astringents
5. Sports and physical activity
   a. Explain that a large water loss may accompany physical activity
   b. Encourage increased water consumption during periods of physical activity to help prevent dehydration
   c. Encourage the adolescent to monitor his weight carefully when in sports training
   d. Point out the importance of a balanced, varied diet with adequate calories to meet increased energy needs
6. Adolescent pregnancy. See Section XII, Nutrition for the Pregnant and Lactating Woman
7. Anorexia nervosa and bulimia
   a. Be aware that adolescent anorexia and bulimia are more common in females
   b. Know the signs and symptoms of eating disorders and teach them to parents and peers: preoccupation with body size or with food, refusal to eat, binge eating, amenorrhea, decreased libido, delayed psychosocial development, compulsive behavior, excessive exercising, poor self-esteem, feelings of depression and anxiety, insomnia, and loss of interest in previously enjoyed activities
   c. Instruct parents in preventive interventions, such as helping the adolescent establish a strong, positive self-image; avoid putting pressure on the adolescent to achieve beyond her capability
   d. Encourage parents to give the adolescent an appropriate amount of independence, responsibility, and accountability for her actions
   e. Teach parents how to recognize stresses in the adolescent's life and provide support and encouragement
   f. Encourage parents to teach the basics of nutrition and normal exercise and to avoid pressuring an obese adolescent to lose weight
   g. Advise the adolescent and parents to seek professional help if eating disorders are suspected

## Points to Remember

Nutritional problems from childhood tend to intensify during adolescence.

Nutritional requirements peak during the years of maximum growth, accompanied by a noticeably increased appetite.

Caloric intake in adolescents should vary to reflect individual growth rates and should balance energy expenditure.

Peer and social pressures and enjoyment tend to exert a greater influence on adolescent food choices than do the nutritional quality of food and the health implications related to diet.

## Glossary

**Acne vulgaris**—skin disorder characterized by eruptions of papules and pustules

**Amenorrhea**—absence of menstruation

**Anorexia nervosa**—emotional disorder characterized by an altered body image, self-imposed starvation, and consequent emaciation

**Bulimia**—obsessive eating (binging) followed by self-induced vomiting or diarrhea (purging) to maintain a desired weight level

**Menstruation**—cyclical process, controlled by hormone levels, that occurs as the lining of the uterus is shed when conception does not occur

# Nutrition for the Adult

## Learning Objectives

After studying this section, the reader should be able to:

• Describe normal physical and psychosocial characteristics of the adult as they relate to nutrition.

• List the nutritional requirements for adults.

• Discuss the nursing implications for promoting healthful nutrition during adulthood.

• Discuss the nursing implications for common nutrition-related problems affecting adults.

# XVII. Nutrition for the Adult

## A. Introduction

1. During *early adulthood*—defined as the period from ages 18 to 40—psychosocial development continues. Major milestones, such as establishing a career and beginning a family, occur at different ages for different people and may greatly influence dietary patterns
2. In *middle adulthood*—between ages 40 and 65—such chronic disorders as heart disease and gouty arthritis may occur, resulting in altered nutritional requirements or food restrictions
3. Available data on food behavior and nutritional needs during adulthood are limited

## B. Normal growth and development

1. Physical characteristics
   a. Physical growth ceases during early adulthood
   b. Signs of aging begin to appear during middle adulthood
2. Psychosocial characteristics
   a. As a young adult becomes more independent, he typically becomes responsible for his own menu planning, food shopping, and meal preparation. This process is easier if the person has learned some basic food preparation and menu planning before leaving his parents' home
   b. The transition to middle adulthood is marked by awareness of the physical changes that signify the beginning of another stage in life; during this period, the adult may reappraise his life and become more concerned about maintaining health

## C. Nutritional requirements

1. General information
   a. Nutritional requirements remain stable throughout adulthood—except for iron requirements
   b. Amounts of specific nutrients decrease from levels that support growth during childhood and adolescence to levels that maintain health
2. Energy (calories)
   a. As adulthood progresses, a decline in physical activity and a slowing of the basal metabolic rate (BMR) decrease caloric requirements
   b. See Appendix A for recommended dietary allowances (RDAs)
3. Protein
   a. Requirements remain relatively stable throughout adulthood
   b. Requirements are higher for men than for women
   c. See Appendix A for RDAs
4. Lipids
   a. No age-specific requirements have been established
   b. Current recommendations stress limiting intake of saturated fats and cholesterol (See Section XI, Dietary Guidelines)

5. Carbohydrates
   a. No age-specific requirements have been established
   b. Recommended levels vary depending on the individual's caloric requirements (See Section XI, Dietary Guidelines)
6. Vitamins
   a. Requirements remain relatively stable throughout adulthood
   b. See Appendix A for RDAs
7. Minerals
   a. Women have an increased need for iron until menopause, after which requirements decrease
   b. Research suggests that a woman's dietary calcium requirements increase after menopause. The recommended daily calcium intake for premenopausal and estrogen-treated postmenopausal women is 1,000 mg; for postmenopausal women, 1,500 mg
8. Fluids
   a. No age-specific requirements have been established
   b. The suggested water intake for an adult is five to eight 8-oz glasses daily, with the specific amount depending on activity level and health status

## D. Promoting healthful nutrition in adults

1. General information
   a. Life-style will influence an adult's food habits and nutritional requirements
   b. The addition of children to the family may focus attention on diet and nutrition
2. Nursing implications: Teach the adult to
   a. Direct his efforts toward developing a healthy life-style by maintaining a diet that meets nutritional needs and by establishing a regular exercise program
   b. Avoid excessive calories, fat, sodium, and sugar
   c. Increase intake of fiber and cruciferous vegetables
   d. Maintain regular dental care to reduce the risk of tooth loss
   e. Avoid using cigarettes or chewing tobacco
   f. Avoid excessive use of alcohol
   g. Take the time to attend to health needs and problems

## E. Nursing implications for common nutrition-related problems of early and middle adulthood

1. Use of birth control methods: the intrauterine device (IUD) and oral contraceptive agents (OCAs)
   a. For a client using an IUD: Monitor for blood loss, which can result in iron deficiency; encourage increased intake of high-iron foods; monitor for iron deficiency anemia; suggest use of an iron supplement or another method of birth control after checking with a physician

b. For a client using OCAs: Explain that OCAs may alter a woman's need for vitamins and minerals; monitor for nutritional deficiencies, particularly Vitamin C, $B_{12}$, riboflavin, pyridoxine, and folic acid; advise the client that becoming pregnant within 6 months of discontinuing OCAs could pose a nutritional risk for both the mother and the fetus

2. Weight gain
   a. Explain why caloric requirements decrease with age and point out that without a balance between caloric intake and use (usually related to regular exercise), weight will increase
   b. Encourage reduction of caloric intake in a nutritionally sound manner
   c. Encourage participation in a regular exercise program
   d. Discourage the use of food as the focus of social relationships
   e. Point out that loneliness and depression often lead to overeating
   f. Offer suggestions on how to avoid overeating
   g. Encourage use of support groups to help with weight loss and weight maintenance

3. Heartburn
   a. Encourage avoidance of caffeine and high-fat foods
   b. Suggest frequent small meals
   c. Evaluate the client's diet and suggest elimination of apparent problem foods
   d. Caution against overusing antacids, which can interfere with iron absorption and may also cause diarrhea or constipation

4. Constipation
   a. Assess for possible causative factors, including irregular bowel habits, psychogenic factors, inactivity, chronic laxative use, inadequate fluid or fiber intake, metabolic or endocrine disorders, bowel abnormalities, or use of certain drugs such as narcotic analgesics
   b. Encourage regular bowel habits
   c. Discourage overuse of laxatives
   d. Suggest drinking hot coffee, tea, or lemon water after waking to stimulate peristalsis
   e. Encourage adequate intake of dietary fiber
   f. Encourage participation in a regular exercise program
   g. Encourage increased fluid intake (if not contraindicated), especially when increasing fiber intake

5. Fatigue
   a. Explain measures to help reduce fatigue, such as planned exercise and rest periods
   b. Encourage advance meal preparation to prevent fatigue from interfering with proper eating
   c. Teach the client about high-energy and high-protein foods

6.  Cessation of smoking
    a.  Alert the client to the potential for weight gain from changes in eating habits or more efficient use of calories and nutrients, but encourage him not to let this possibility discourage him from giving up smoking
    b.  Provide guidelines from the American Heart Association, American Lung Association, or American Cancer Society on weight control for former smokers
    c.  Advise using low-calorie beverages and snacks to help resist the craving for cigarettes
7.  Bleeding gums
    a.  Be aware that bleeding gums may result from poor oral hygiene or periodontal disease rather than from vitamin C deficiency
    b.  Promote effective dental hygiene to help prevent gum disease and resulting tooth loss and chewing difficulties
8.  Skeletal changes
    a.  Explain that bone density peaks at age 35 and decreases thereafter; this process is most rapid in postmenopausal women, placing them at risk for osteoporosis
    b.  Stress that prevention of osteoporosis is more effective than treatment
    c.  Encourage adequate dietary calcium intake beginning early in life
    d.  Encourage maintenance of proper weight, with weight reduction as necessary
    e.  Encourage participation in regular weight-bearing exercise to prevent calcium loss from bone
    f.  Suggest that a postmenopausal woman discuss estrogen replacement therapy with her physician

## Points to Remember

As a young adult becomes more independent, he typically becomes responsible for his own menu planning, food shopping, and meal preparation. This process is easier if the person has learned some basic food preparation and menu planning before leaving his parents' home.

The transition to middle adulthood is marked by awareness of the physical changes that signify the beginning of another stage in life; during this period, the adult may reappraise his life and become more concerned about maintaining health.

As adulthood progresses, a decline in physical activity and a slowing of the basal metabolic rate decrease caloric requirements.

Unbalanced caloric intake and use usually lead to weight gain during adulthood.

## Glossary

**Menopause**—period during which a woman's menstrual cycle wanes and gradually ceases

**Oral contraceptive agent**—pharmacologic agent taken by mouth that prevents pregnancy by inhibiting ovulation

**Osteoporosis**—metabolic bone disorder marked by increased bone resorption and decreased bone formation, resulting in a loss of bone mass

**Periodontal disease**—degenerative process that undermines supporting structures of the teeth

# Nutrition for the Older Adult

**Learning Objectives**

After studying this section, the reader should be able to:

• Describe the normal physical and psychosocial characteristics for the older adult as they relate to nutrition.

• List the nutritional requirements for the older adult.

• Discuss the nursing implications for promoting healthful nutrition in the older adult.

• Discuss the nursing implications for common nutrition-related problems affecting the older adult.

# XVIII. Nutrition for the Older Adult

## A.  Introduction

1.  An older adult is defined as a person age 60 or older
2.  Nutrition plays an important, though as-yet imprecisely defined, role in the aging process
3.  Following sound nutritional practices throughout life increases a person's chance of maintaining good health as aging occurs
4.  Various physiologic, psychosocial, and economic factors may increase an older person's vulnerability to nutritional problems
5.  Common dietary deficiencies affecting the older adult include protein, vitamin C, vitamin D, folic acid, calcium, and iron

## B.  Normal growth and development

1.  Physical characteristics
    a.  The rate of aging varies widely among individuals
    b.  Within an individual, organs and body systems may age at widely varying rates
    c.  The age-related decline in functional capacity of most body organs and systems is least apparent when the organ or system is in a resting state, and most apparent when it is stressed
    d.  Lean body mass gradually diminishes, accompanied by an increase in adipose and fibrous connective tissues
    e.  Basal metabolic rate declines about 16% from ages 30 to 70; as a result, an aging person requires fewer calories to maintain body weight
    f.  Sensory changes include partial loss of taste and smell and deterioration of sight and hearing
    g.  Changes in the buccal cavity include a high incidence of tooth loss, reduction in saliva output to approximately ⅓ the volume of earlier years, decreased salivary ptyalin levels, and atrophy of oral mucosal epithelium
    h.  GI changes include diminished gag reflex, decreased esophageal peristalsis and increased relaxation of the lower esophageal sphincter, decreased stomach motility, decreased secretion of hydrochloric acid and pepsin, slowed gastric emptying time, decreased fat tolerance, less efficient cholesterol stabilization and absorption, increased fat content of the pancreas, decreased pancreatic enzyme levels, decreased colonic peristalsis, and diminished sensation of the need to defecate
    i.  Kidney function changes include altered ability to dilute and concentrate urine, and decreased efficiency in removing body wastes
2.  Psychosocial characteristics: an older adult who cannot accept changes related to aging may develop nutritional problems from lack of variety in diet and disinterest in food
    a.  Adjusting to decreasing health and physical strength
    b.  Adjusting to retirement and reduced income
    c.  Adjusting to the death of a spouse
    d.  Accepting oneself as an aging person

    e. Maintaining satisfactory living arrangements
    f. Realigning relationships with adult children
    g. Finding meaning in life

## C. Nutritional requirements

1. General information
   a. Food intake is generally less, whether because of a natural result of aging or psychosocial changes
   b. No standard recommendations for nutrients for adults over age 65 have been established
   c. Recommended dietary requirements (RDAs) are based on the general population over age 51
2. Energy (calories)
   a. With aging comes a decrease in the body's rate of energy consumption and, consequently, in caloric requirements
   b. See Appendix A for RDAs for clients ages 51 to 75
   c. The RDA for men ages 76 and older ranges from 1,650 to 2,450 calories per day; for women ages 76 and older, from 1,200 to 2,000 calories per day
3. Protein
   a. Controversy exists over the requirements for healthy older adults
   b. Adequate protein intake is necessary to prevent excessive loss of muscle tissue
   c. See Appendix A for RDAs
4. Lipids. No age-specific recommendations have been established
5. Carbohydrates
   a. Many authorities recommend increased intake of complex carbohydrates, which generally provide fewer calories than refined carbohydrates
   b. Increased dietary fiber intake may help prevent problems associated with decreased GI motility and may help reduce the risk of GI cancer
6. Vitamins
   a. An older adult's vitamin requirements remain essentially the same as those for a younger adult
   b. An older adult is more susceptible to vitamin deficiencies from low dietary intake or diseases that reduce absorption or stores of vitamins than a younger adult
   c. Chronic use of certain drugs may accentuate some deficient states
   d. Symptoms of deficiency may be vague and masked by other disorders or by adverse drug reactions
   e. Low-potency vitamin supplements may be required in a person with a total daily caloric intake of 1,500 or less
   f. See Appendix A for RDAs
7. Minerals
   a. Dietary mineral intake is usually adequate unless diet is severely restricted

b. Decreased gastric secretions may result in decreased absorption of iron and calcium

c. As a result, an older adult may need supplements to prevent iron deficiency anemia and decrease the risk of osteoporosis

d. See Appendix A for RDAs

8. Fluids

a. An older adult is susceptible to both overhydration and dehydration

b. Factors that may cause an older adult to restrict fluids include decreased sensation of thirst, lack of motivation, fear of incontinence or nocturia, inaccessibility of fluids, inability to drink without assistance, and altered mental status

c. Fluid restriction may lead to infection, constipation, decreased bladder capacity, and fluid and electrolyte imbalances

d. Fluid excess problems are usually related to decreased cardiovascular and renal function

e. Recommended fluid intake ranges from 2,500 to 3,000 ml/day

**D. Promoting healthful nutrition in the older adult**

1. General information

a. An older adult may be at risk for poor nutrition

b. Any new or additional stress can have serious nutritional implications

c. Good nutrition improves the prognosis in any illness or injury

2. Nursing implications: Encourage the older adult to

a. Select nutrient-rich, relatively low-fat foods

b. Keep serving sizes small to accommodate changes in the GI tract

c. Ingest plenty of water and other fluids to maintain adequate hydration and promote good bowel function

d. Avoid excessive salt intake to reduce fluid retention and help prevent hypertension

e. Experiment with new seasoning methods to reduce salt intake

f. Avoid relying totally on convenience foods and canned goods, which typically contain high levels of salt and preservatives

g. Adjust food preparation methods to accommodate any chewing problems

h. Follow any prescribed diet modifications

i. Share cooking responsibilities with others, if possible

j. Make arrangements to eat at least several meals per week with friends, neighbors, or relatives, if possible

k. Use available money-saving resources and community services, such as federal food stamps, Meals On Wheels, free bus service to local supermarkets, and senior citizen centers

l. Participate in physical activities as appropriate

**E. Nursing implications for common nutrition-related problems affecting the older adult**

1. Alcohol abuse

a. Be aware that an older adult may turn to alcohol to combat feelings of loneliness, social isolation, and despair

   b. Encourage participation in outside activities, such as those available through local senior citizen centers
   c. Explain that overuse of alcohol can eventually result in reduced food intake, possibly leading to malnutrition
   d. Evaluate dietary patterns; offer suggestions to enhance nutritional intake and discourage alcohol use
2. Mental status changes
   a. Evaluate level of consciousness and ability to recall dietary intake
   b. As appropriate, arrange for a companion, friend, neighbor, relative, or home health aide to help with meal preparation and eating
   c. Arrange for Meals On Wheels, if available and necessary
   d. Provide written reminders of when and what to eat
   e. Continually assess the client's ability to obtain adequate nutrition, and notify the physician of any significant changes
3. Chronic diseases
   a. Evaluate the disease's effect on the client's nutritional status
   b. Assess for disease-related factors affecting nutrient intake, such as dietary modifications, interactions between foods and drugs, and limited mobility
   c. Assist the client in disease management
   d. Help the client understand and comply with any prescribed dietary restrictions; offer suggestions and alternatives for food selection and preparation
4. Dehydration
   a. Assess for signs and symptoms, including dry, inelastic skin; dry, brown tongue; sunken cheeks and eyeballs; concentrated urine; and possibly confusion
   b. Carefully monitor intake and output and body weight
   c. Encourage fluid intake of at least 2,500 ml/day (if not contraindicated)
   d. Teach the client about alternate sources of fluids, such as ice cream, pudding, and gelatin desserts
5. Anorexia
   a. Assess dietary intake, and evaluate for possible causes of anorexia →
   b. Encourage the client to eat small, frequent meals
   c. Suggest that the client try to stimulate interest in meals by setting an attractive table, preparing colorful foods, and eating with a companion
   d. Check weight frequently
   e. Explain the advantages and disadvantages of taking vitamin and mineral supplements
6. Constipation
   a. Evaluate dietary intake and bowel elimination patterns
   b. Check medication history for possible causative factors
   c. Encourage increased intake of high-fiber foods
   d. Encourage increased fluid intake (if not contraindicated)
   e. Encourage regular exercise, such as walking, to enhance peristalsis

## Points to Remember

Nutrition plays an important, though as-yet imprecisely defined, role in the aging process.

Following sound nutritional practices throughout life increases an older adult's chances of maintaining good health.

Various physiologic, psychosocial, and economic factors often increase an older adult's vulnerability to nutritional problems.

Common dietary deficiencies affecting older adults include protein, vitamin C, vitamin D, folic acid, calcium, and iron.

## Glossary

**Nocturia**—excessive urination at night

**Urinary incontinence**—inability to control urination

# Nutrition and the Nursing Process

## Learning Objectives

After studying this section, the reader should be able to:

- Discuss the collection and use of nutritional data as part of the nursing process.

- Discuss the role of nursing diagnosis in providing nutritional care to a client.

- Identify the general nursing interventions for providing nutritional care.

- Identify examples of outcome criteria used in evaluating nutritional care.

- List possible nursing interventions after problem identification.

- Discuss possible nursing interventions for common nutrition-related problems of hospitalized clients.

- Identify support services available for clients with nutritional problems.

# XIX. Nutrition and the Nursing Process

## A. Introduction
1. Goals
   a. Identify actual or potential nutritional needs
   b. Establish plans to meet these nutritional needs
   c. Perform specific nursing interventions to meet nutritional needs
2. General nursing interventions for providing nutritional care
   a. Assess the client's nutritional status
   b. Evaluate the client's risk for nutritional problems
   c. Observe the client's nutritional intake
   d. Provide nutritional care in a systematic manner, using the nursing process
   e. Consider the many factors that affect the client's food choices
   f. Act as part of the health care team responsible for nutritional care

## B. Assessment
1. Purpose: To develop a baseline of information for problem identification and core planning
2. Aids in identifying
   a. Overt malnutrition
   b. Covert malnutrition
   c. Clients at risk for developing malnutrition
   d. Clients at risk for developing nutrition-related diseases
   e. Resources to help clients overcome nutritional problems
   f. Client's nutritional status and requirements for maintenance, growth, or repletion of body tissue
3. Components of a nutritional assessment
   a. Dietary history
   b. Clinical assessment data collection
   c. Anthropometric measurements
   d. Diagnostic test findings

## C. Diagnosis
1. Purpose: To identify client problems
2. Accomplished through identifying nursing diagnoses specific to the actual or potential nutritional problem; for example,
   a. Alteration in nutritional status: less than body requirements
   b. Alteration in nutritional status: greater than body requirements
   c. Impaired swallowing
   d. Self-care deficit
   e. Disturbance in self-care concept
   f. Alteration in fluid volume: excess
   g. Alteration in fluid volume: deficit
   h. Impaired social interaction
   i. Alteration in growth and development

3. Accomplished through identification of collaborative problems by the nurse and the multidisciplinary team for definitive treatment; for example,
   a. Potential alteration in fluid and electrolyte balance
   b. Potential cardiac dysrhythmias
   c. Potential GI disturbances, such as hemorrhage

## D. Planning
1. Purpose: To plan nutritional interventions and establish outcome criteria
2. Accomplished through choosing nursing interventions that will ameliorate the problem and through organizing client care into a comprehensive nursing care plan

## E. Implementation
1. Purpose: To carry out planned nursing interventions after problem identification
2. Nursing interventions related to nutritional care
   a. Providing health teaching to the client and family regarding the importance of a balanced, nutritious diet throughout life; regular mealtimes; avoidance of emotional stress before, during, and after meals; proper dental care and oral hygiene; periodic health evaluation; and a regular and balanced exercise program
   b. Providing patient teaching about dietary instructions
   c. Providing nutritional therapy by using an optimum diet for each client. Types of diets include normal diets, special diets, therapeutic diets, enteral therapy, and parenteral therapy
   d. Checking and confirming the physician's diet orders and ensuring that the client receives the proper diet tray by checking the tray for client's name, type of diet, and completeness of tray
   e. Providing any prescribed medications before, during, or after meals, as indicated, to prevent or minimize possible adverse reactions
   f. Ensuring proper hand washing, oral hygiene, and elimination before and after meals
   g. Ensuring a comfortable and safe position for eating
   h. Preparing the diet tray to meet the client's needs by opening cartons, cutting foods, and seasoning foods, as necessary
   i. Providing special eating utensils
   j. Allowing the client to make food choices, as appropriate
   k. Monitoring and documenting the client's dietary intake and tolerance
   l. Consulting with other health care professionals, as necessary, to modify the client's diet or take other measures to improve the client's nutritional status
   m. Assisting the client with changing eating behaviors, if necessary

## F. Evaluation
1. Purpose: To determine the client's response to nutritional therapy and nursing interventions based on the outcome criteria established in the planning phase

2. Accomplished through outcome criteria related to nutritional status and nutrient intake; for example,
   a. The client will have a tricep skinfold measurement within the predetermined acceptable range
   b. The client will have a stable daily weight
   c. The client will maintain fluid intake at the prescribed level
   d. The client will achieve the planned weekly weight loss while on a weight-reduction diet
   e. The client will feed himself independently using self-feeding aids, if necessary
   f. The client will eat an entire meal without feeling nauseated
   g. The client will plan a balanced meal using the dietary information provided
   h. The client will identify foods high in potassium

## G. Nursing implications for common nutrition-related problems of hospitalized clients

1. Anorexia
   a. Assess for possible causative factors, such as limited physical activity or poor oral hygiene, and reduce or eliminate these factors as appropriate
   b. Relieve illness symptoms that contribute to decreased appetite
   c. Provide food preferred by the client, as possible
   d. Provide a pleasant environment during mealtimes to help enhance interest in eating
   e. Reduce any sources of emotional stress that may decrease appetite
2. Nausea or vomiting
   a. Assess for possible causative factors, such as obnoxious odors, and reduce or eliminate these factors as appropriate
   b. Instruct the client to eat and drink slowly
   c. Provide small, frequent meals rather than large meals to decrease feelings of fullness
   d. Encourage the client to drink fluids between meals rather than with meals
   e. Instruct the client to avoid poorly tolerated foods, highly acidic foods, and foods high in fat
   f. Encourage the client to rest for an hour or more following a meal
   g. Provide dry toast or crackers when the client feels nauseated
   h. Teach the client to relax, take deep breaths, and swallow when nauseated
   i. Provide prescribed antacids or antiemetics as directed to decrease GI symptoms
3. Mild diarrhea
   a. Assess for possible causative factors, such as excessive dietary fiber intake, and reduce or eliminate these factors as appropriate
   b. Limit intake initially to liquids, gradually adding solids as the client can tolerate them

    c. Instruct the client to avoid milk and milk products, extremely hot or cold food, and concentrated sweets, all of which may aggravate diarrhea

    d. Provide soft foods that contain pectin, such as bananas and applesauce, to promote intestinal water absorption and thereby decrease diarrhea

    e. Provide low-fiber foods to decrease bowel motility

    f. Promote relaxation techniques

    g. Provide prescribed antispasmodics and antidiarrheals as directed to decrease GI symptoms

4. Constipation

    a. Assess for possible causative factors, such as inadequate fluid intake, and reduce or eliminate these factors as appropriate

    b. Help the client establish a consistent pattern of food intake and elimination

    c. Encourage the client to eat breakfast or at least drink a hot beverage on arising in the morning to stimulate peristalsis

    d. Provide foods high in dietary fiber, such as bran cereals, to promote elimination

    e. Provide foods that act as natural laxatives, such as prunes

    f. Ensure adequate fluid intake (at least 1,000 ml/day) if the client isn't fluid-restricted

    g. Teach the client to establish a pattern of regular physical activity

    h. Teach the client to avoid overusing laxatives and explain that reliance on laxatives suppresses normal bowel activity, thus promoting constipation

5. Flatus

    a. Instruct the client to avoid foods and eating-related behaviors (such as air-swallowing) that may produce gas

    b. Teach the client to avoid reclining immediately after meals

    c. Decrease the fat content of meals to reduce the time food remains in the stomach

6. Fluid restriction

    a. Monitor fluid intake to ensure that it falls within set limits

    b. Be alert for changes in the environment or the client's health status, such as an increase in room temperature or a fever, that might require an adjustment in fluid intake

    c. Consider the client's preferences when selecting fluids

    d. Include fluids used to prepare and administer medications when calculating a client's total fluid intake

    e. Instruct the client to avoid salty or highly sweetened foods, which can cause increased thirst

    f. Divide the daily fluid allotment to ensure sufficient intake throughout the waking hours

7. Fluid increase (forcing fluids)

    a. Consider the client's preferences when selecting fluid sources; alternatives to water include fruit juices, carbonated beverages, broth, gelatin desserts, frozen ice pops, and fruit sherbets

    b. Provide small portions of different fluid sources frequently, rather than large portions infrequently

c. Keep liquids at the client's bedside
d. Advise the physician if the client cannot maintain adequate hydration orally; the client may require I.V. fluids
e. Advise the physician if a client on I.V. fluids is able to obtain adequate hydration orally; the physician may order I.V. fluids discontinued
8. Difficulty chewing
  a. Assess for possible causative factors, such as extensive dental caries or ill-fitting dentures, and reduce or eliminate these factors as appropriate
  b. Provide easily chewed foods of different textures and tastes, ensure that all foods are cooked until tender, and cut food into small pieces
  c. Provide protein and calorie supplements if dietary intake is inadequate
9. Difficulty swallowing
  a. Assess for possible causative factors, such as inappropriate positioning during eating, and reduce or eliminate such factors as appropriate
  b. Before offering fluids or food, assess level of consciousness, gag reflex, and the ability to swallow saliva to prevent aspiration
  c. Keep suction equipment on hand and readily available
  d. Position the client sitting upright with the head flexed forward on midline about 45 degrees to help keep the esophagus patent
  e. Offer small amounts of fluids initially, gradually increasing the amounts in response to the client's tolerance
  f. Feed the client slowly, making certain that he swallows one mouthful of food before offering more
  g. Advise the physician if the client cannot obtain adequate nutrition through oral feeding; the physician may order tube feeding or parental nutrition

## H. Nutritional support services
1. General information
  a. Provide for clients who cannot handle their at-home nutritional needs
  b. Include various governmental and community services that assist people with nutritional needs
  c. Offer referrals for the nurse who is planning care
2. Food Stamp Program
  a. Established by the Food Stamp Act of 1977
  b. Administered by the U.S. Department of Agriculture (USDA)
  c. Provides food stamps for use in purchasing all food items (except pet food and alcoholic beverages) at any grocery store; benefit amount calculated based on family size and income
  d. Aimed to promote good nutrition for the impoverished population
3. Special Supplementary Food Program for Women, Infants, and Children (WIC)
  a. Administered by the USDA's Food and Nutrition Service
  b. Designed to improve the nutritional intake of pregnant and lactating women, infants, and young children who are at high nutritional risk

      c. Provides specific supplemental foods either directly or through vouchers that people can use to purchase designated foods

      d. Requires that the recipient be affiliated with an established health clinic

4. National School Lunch and Breakfast Programs

      a. Resulted from the National School Lunch Act of 1946 and the Child Nutrition Act

      b. Provides qualifying children at participating schools with reduced-price or free meals

5. Nutritional Program for Older Americans

      a. Administered by the U.S. Department of Health and Human Services' Administration on Aging; also known as Title III or congregate meals for elderly people

      b. Requires that a recipient be age 60 or older, or the spouse of someone who is; financial and health status are not considered

      c. Provides community-based noontime meals at least 5 days per week at optional nominal fees; each meal is planned to provide ⅓ of the recommended dietary allowances (RDAs) for a elderly person

      d. Also offers nutritional education and health and welfare counseling

      e. Provides the added benefit of allowing recurring social interaction with others

6. Meals On Wheels

      a. Sponsored by local community volunteer agencies

      b. Designed for elderly people who cannot prepare meals or leave their homes

      c. Provides ready-to-eat or frozen dinners, with fees based on a sliding scale according to the person's ability to pay

7. Grocery delivery services: Provided by local community agencies for people who are unable to shop for groceries

8. Food Distribution Program (Commodity Assistance)

      a. Administered by the USDA

      b. Provides food primarily for programs such as School Lunch and Breakfast and Title III, and for local charitable institutions

      c. Consists of donated foods, such as frozen turkey and chicken, canned applesauce, peanut butter, and cheese, usually acquired under price support and surplus removal legislation

9. Health maintenance programs

      a. Established by many businesses for their employees

      b. Generally include exercise facilities, stress reduction programs, and nutritional counseling

10. Volunteer health agencies

      a. Provide nutrition and diet consultation and nutrition educational materials

      b. Include agencies such as the American Heart Association (AHA), American Diabetes Association (ADA), and American Cancer Society (ACS)

## Points to Remember

To provide optimum nutritional care, the nurse first assesses the client's nutritional needs, then develops and implements a nutritional care plan, and finally evaluates and documents the client's response.

Nutrition-related nursing interventions involve client counseling about nutrition, referring clients to community-based nutritional services, and providing nutritional therapy and specific nursing interventions aimed at dealing with nutritional problems.

A nurse can improve a client's nutritional intake by evaluating the client and his environment before meals are served.

Many nutrition-related problems of hospitalized clients can be alleviated through nursing interventions.

## Glossary

**Anthropometric measurements**—scientific measurements of various body dimensions

**Antiemetic**—agent that prevents or relieves nausea and vomiting

**Collaborative problem**—physiologic condition or complication that results or may result from a pathophysiologic- or treatment-related situation; falls within the domains of medicine and nursing, amenable primarily to medical interventions; the nurse does not treat the problem independently but may initiate its monitoring

**Nursing process**—systematic, rational method of planning and providing nursing care that encompasses four steps: assessment, planning, implementation, and evaluation

# Nutritional Assessment

## Learning Objectives

After studying this section, the reader should be able to:

- List the steps used in obtaining a nutritional assessment.

- Describe the data used in nutritional assessment.

- Explain the major goals of nutritional assessment.

- List factors that can put a client at risk for nutritional problems.

- Describe the general characteristics and nursing implications of a dietary history.

- Describe the use of anthropometric measurements in nutritional assessment.

- Describe the most common diagnostic studies used in nutritional assessment.

## XX. Nutritional Assessment

### A. Introduction

1. Nutritional assessment involves collecting data to establish a client's nutritional status
2. Steps of nutritional assessment
   a. Obtaining a nursing health history related to nutritional status
   b. Performing a physical assessment
   c. Reviewing pertinent laboratory test results and other records related to nutrition
   d. Consulting with other health team members, such as dietitians
   e. Reviewing current literature related to nutritional care
3. Types of data involved in nutritional assessment
   a. Subjective data—information provided by the client in the health history interview
   b. Objective data—information obtained by the nurse through physical assessment and evaluation of laboratory test results and other records
4. Components of a nutritional assessment
   a. Dietary history
   b. Clinical assessment data collection
   c. Anthropometric measurements
   d. Diagnostic studies
5. Goals of nutritional assessment
   a. Determining the client's actual or potential nutritional status resulting from the intake and use of essential nutrients
   b. Identifying and determining the cause of any actual or potential nutritional problem
   c. Providing baseline data from which a nursing diagnosis can be developed
   d. Providing a plan for implementing ongoing interventions that alleviate nutritional problems
6. Factors increasing a client's risk for nutritional problems
   a. Usual body weight 20% above or below normal standards
   b. Recent loss or gain of 10% of usual body weight
   c. Inadequate food intake, food budget, or food preparation facilities
   d. Chewing or swallowing difficulties
   e. Excessive use of alcohol
   f. Frequent use of fad diets or monotonous diets
   g. Living alone and preparing own meals
   h. No oral intake other than simple fluids for 10 or more days
   i. GI surgery, other than appendectomy
   j. Recent major surgery, illness, or injury
   k. History of diabetes, hypertension, hyperlipidemia, coronary artery disease, malabsorption syndrome, circulatory problems or heart failure, neurologic disorder or paralysis, mental disability, teenage pregnancy, multiple pregnancy, cancer, radiation therapy, or chronic lung, renal, or liver disease

    l.   History of certain medication use, such as catabolic steroids, immunosuppressants, antitumor agents, oral contraceptives, antibiotics, antacids, antidepressants, antihypertensives, digitalis, laxatives, diuretics, potassium chloride, vitamin and other nutrient preparations, anticonvulsants, and anti-inflammatory agents

7.   Poor nutritional status affects most body systems; assessment of body systems can sometimes reveal nutritional problems

8.   Clinical signs of poor nutrition may be observable only in clients with long-standing nutritional problems; most clinical signs of nutritional deficiency that nurses typically see are mild and nonspecific

9.   Signs and symptoms of healthful nutrition
   a. Alertness and responsiveness, with a good attention span and no signs of irritability or restlessness
   b. Normal weight for height, age, and body build
   c. Erect posture and straight arms and legs, with well-developed, firm muscles and some subcutaneous fat; no skeletal malformations
   d. Normal reflexes
   e. Good appetite and digestion with normal, regular elimination pattern and no palpable abdominal masses
   f. Normal heart rate and rhythm, with no murmurs, and normal blood pressure for age
   g. Good energy level and no reported sleeping problems
   h. Shiny, lustrous, firmly rooted hair and a healthy scalp
   i. Smooth, slightly moist skin with uniform, healthy color
   j. Smooth, moist lips with good color, with no chapping or swelling
   k. Reddish-pink, healthy-looking oral mucosa
   l. Pink gums with no swelling or bleeding
   m. Reddish pink tongue, not swollen or smooth, surface papillae present with no lesions
   n. Clean, nondiscolored teeth, with no pain or caries
   o. Bright, clear, shiny eyes with no sores at corners of eyelids; moist, pink conjunctival membranes with no prominent blood vessels or tissue mounds; no fatigue circles beneath the eyes
   p. Normal size neck, with no enlargement or masses
   q. Firm, pink nails
   r. No tenderness, weakness, swelling, or discoloration in the legs or feet

10.   Signs and symptoms of poor nutrition (See *Nutritional disorders: An assessment guide* for more information)
   a. Listlessness, apathy, inattentiveness, irritability, or confusion
   b. Overweight or underweight for height and body frame
   c. Poor posture with sagging shoulders, sunken chest, or humped back; flaccid, poorly developed, weak, or tender muscles; skeletal deformities such as bowlegs, knock-knees, chest deformity at diaphragm, beaded ribs, and prominent scapulae

# NUTRITIONAL DISORDERS: AN ASSESSMENT GUIDE

| BODY SYSTEM OR REGION | SIGN OR SYMPTOM | IMPLICATIONS |
|---|---|---|
| General | Weakness, fatigue | Electrolyte imbalance, anemia, hypophosphatemia |
| | Weight loss | Marked calorie intake reduction or increased calorie use; decreased fat, protein, or carbohydrate absorption |
| | Edema | Protein deficiency |
| Integumentary | Anemia (pallor) | Iron, vitamin $B_{12}$, or folic acid deficiency |
| | Dry skin and mucous membranes, poor skin turgor | Dehydration |
| | Dermatitis | Niacin, riboflavin, pyridoxine, zinc, or fatty acid (for example, linoleic acid) deficiency |
| | Rough, scaly skin with hard papillae at hair follicle bases | Vitamin A deficiency |
| | Ecchymoses, hemorrhagic tendency | Vitamin K deficiency (inhibits production of clotting Factors II, VII, IX, and X), ascorbic acid deficiency |
| | Spoon-shaped, brittle, or ridged nails | Iron deficiency |
| | Hair thinning, loss, or dryness | Protein or copper deficiency |
| | Decubitus ulcers | Protein-calorie deficiency |
| | Sores that don't heal | Protein, vitamin C, or zinc deficiency |
| | Petechiae | Vitamin C deficiency |
| | Xanthomas | Increased serum low-density lipoprotein or very-low-density lipoprotein levels, with resultant hyperlipoproteinemia |
| Head, eye, ear, nose, and throat | Night blindness, corneal dryness, eyelid swelling | Vitamin A deficiency |
| | Increased sensitivity to bright light; burning, itching, or sore eyes | Vitamin A or riboflavin deficiency |
| | Dark circles under eyes | Vitamin B complex (especially niacin) deficiency |

continued

From *Metabolic Problems*. NurseReview series. Springhouse, Pa.: Springhouse Corp., 1988, pp. 26-27.

## NUTRITIONAL DISORDERS: AN ASSESSMENT GUIDE continued

| BODY SYSTEM OR REGION | SIGN OR SYMPTOM | IMPLICATIONS |
|---|---|---|
| Head, eye, ear, nose, and throat (continued) | Glossitis | Vitamin $B_{12}$ or C, folic acid, iron, riboflavin, pyridoxine, cyanocobalamin, or niacin deficiency |
| | Cheilosis (cracks at corner of mouth) | Riboflavin, niacin, pyridoxine, or iron deficiency |
| | Dental decay | Calcium, phosphorus, fluoride, or vitamin A or D deficiency; excess sucrose intake |
| | Soft, spongy, bleeding gums | Vitamin C deficiency |
| | Simple goiter | Iodine deficiency |
| Cardiovascular | Hypotension | Dehydration |
| | Tachycardia | Hypovolemia, anemia |
| | Peripheral edema | Protein malabsorption or enteric protein loss |
| Gastrointestinal | Diarrhea, flatulence, borborygmi, distention | Impaired water, sodium, fatty acid, bile, or carbohydrate absorption |
| | Ascites | Hypoproteinemia |
| | Malodorous, greasy stools | Steatorrhea |
| | Loss of taste | Protein or zinc deficiency |
| Musculoskeletal | Bone pain | Vitamin D deficiency, hypocalcemia, hypophosphatemia |
| | Muscle cramps | Hypokalemia |
| | Muscle wasting | Protein malabsorption, reduced carbohydrate and fat sources for metabolic energy |
| | Bowlegs, knock-knee, chest deformity, beaded ribs, prominent scapulae | Vitamin D, calcium, or phosphorus deficiency |
| Neurologic | Altered mental state | Dehydration, vitamin $B_{12}$ deficiency |
| | Paresthesias, ataxia | Vitamin $B_{12}$, pyridoxine, or thiamine deficiency |
| | Tetany, Chvostek's or Trousseau's sign | Hypocalcemia, hypomagnesemia, vitamin D deficiency |
| Genitourinary | Genital rash | Zinc deficiency |

  d.  Burning and tingling of the hands and feet, loss of position and vibratory sense, decreased or absent ankle and knee reflexes
  e.  Anorexia, indigestion, constipation or diarrhea, liver or spleen enlargement
  f.  Rapid heart rate, enlarged heart, abnormal cardiac rhythm, elevated blood pressure
  g.  Low energy level, easy fatigability, cachexia
  h.  Dull, brittle, dry, thin, depigmented, and easily plucked hair
  i.  Rough, dry, scaly, pale or irregularly pigmented skin with areas of irritation, bruising, or petechiae
  j.  Dry, scaly, swollen lips with fissures or scars and possibly redness and swelling or lesions at the corners of the mouth
  k.  Swollen, boggy oral mucous membranes
  l.  Spongy, bleeding, inflamed, or receding gums
  m. Swollen, scarlet or magenta, raw, beefy, hyperemic tongue with atrophic or hypertrophic papillae
  n.  Decayed, absent, worn, mottled, or malpositioned teeth
  o.  Pale or inflamed conjunctival membranes; signs of infection; redness and fissuring of eyelid corners; dull, soft corneas
  p.  Enlarged thyroid
  q.  Spoon-shaped, brittle, ridged nails
  r.  Edema, tenderness, tingling, and weakness in the legs and feet
11. General factors affecting dietary patterns
  a.  Cultural background
  b.  Religion
  c.  Life-style
  d.  Personal preferences
  e.  Economic status
  f.  Peer group influences
  g.  Advertising influences
  h.  Psychological factors
  i.  Health status
  j.  Alcohol and drug use
  k.  Age and developmental stage
  l.  Misinformation and food fads

## B. Dietary history
1. General information
  a.  A dietary history involves an evaluation of the nutritional adequacy of the client's diet
  b.  A dietary history is a summary of major factors affecting food intake, such as how much and when the client eats
2. Purposes
  a.  To identify actual or potential nutritional problems
  b.  To identify causes of nutritional problems
  c.  To serve as a useful foundation for nutritional interventions

3. Nursing implications
   a. Explain to the client the type of dietary history to be used (for example, 24-hour recall or food diary) and what information he will need to supply
   b. Be aware that the client may be unwilling to share information truthfully and may overreport small intakes and underreport large intakes
   c. Try to ask open-ended questions
   d. Provide models of food servings and measuring cups and spoons to help the client estimate quantities
   e. Analyze the client's diet by comparing the results of his dietary recall with his actual nutritional requirements using appropriate guidelines
   f. Determine broad areas of dietary weaknesses

C. **Anthropometry**
   1. General information
      a. Anthropometry is an objective, noninvasive method of measuring overall body size and composition as well as specific body parts
      b. Measurements are relatively quick, easy, and inexpensive to perform
      c. Anthropmetric data can reflect long-term changes in nutritional intake
      d. These data must be evaluated according to appropriate reference standards for the client's age and sex
   2. Purposes
      a. To evaluate nutritional status
      b. To monitor growth and development in children
      c. To monitor effects of nutritional interventions
   3. Potential problems
      a. Errors in measurement may result from an examiner's inexperience, an uncooperative client, or inaccurate equipment
      b. Significant changes in nutritional status, such as changes in anthropometric measurements, may manifest themselves slowly in adults
      c. Height and weight may be altered by disease conditions, such as osteoporosis or edema, thus reflecting information not related to nutritional status
      d. Reference standards may not be appropriate for all populations
   4. Types
      a. Weight
      b. Height
      c. Ideal body weight
      d. Body frame size
      e. Mid-arm circumference
      f. Skinfold thickness
      g. Mid-arm muscle circumference

## D. Weight
1. General information (See Appendix D for height and weight tables.)
   a. Weight is the most commonly recorded anthropometric measurement
   b. It reflects the total weight of lean body mass and fat
   c. The current standards of ideal body weight are based on Society of Actuaries data
   d. The procedure requires a calibrated, upright balance beam scale; bed scale if client is bedridden; or pediatric scale if client is an infant
   e. Weight should be measured to nearest ¼ lb (0.1 kg) and recorded, then compared to appropriate reference standard and to previous measurement
2. Purposes
   a. To determine whether a client's weight is appropriate for his height
   b. To detect weight loss or gain
3. Interpretation of data
   a. Normal values: within 10% above or below the recommended weight
   b. Overweight: 10% to 20% above recommended weight
   c. Obese: 20% or more above recommended weight
   d. Underweight: 10% to 20% below recommended weight
   e. Seriously underweight: 20% or more below recommended weight

## E. Height
1. General information (See Appendix D for height and weight tables.)
   a. To measure a client's height, the client must be able to stand without assistance
   b. Height is usually recorded for a child ages 2 to 3 who is able to stand unassisted; infants are measured in the recumbent position and the measurement is recorded as length
   c. The procedure requires a measuring stick or nonstretchable measuring tape attached to a flat, vertical surface, and a movable headpiece that forms a right angle to the vertical surface
   d. A movable measuring rod on an upright balance beam scale provides accurate measurements only when it maintains a parallel position to the floor and rests securely on the topmost part of the crown of the head
   e. Height should be measured to the nearest ⅛" (0.3 cm) and recorded, then compared to appropriate reference standards and to previous measurements
2. Purposes
   a. To determine whether a child's height is within the normal range for his developmental stage
   b. To detect growth deficiency, a possible sign of chronic undernutrition in children
   c. To identify changes in bone and body composition of adults
3. Interpretation of data
   a. Child: height at 5th percentile or below for age indicates a risk of growth retardation or stunting
   b. Adult: height typically decreases with advancing age over 60 years

**F. Ideal body weight (IBW)**
1. General information
   a. IBW compares the client's weight with reference-standard weight values for given heights
   b. IBW is expressed as a percentage, calculated by dividing actual body weight by ideal body weight (reference-standard values), then multiplying this figure by 100
   c. The reference standards of weight-to-height are controversial
   d. The most commonly used standards are those published by the Metropolitan Life Company; these standards are based on weights associated with the lowest mortality rate for persons between ages 25 and 59, and allow for differences in body frame size
2. Purposes
   a. To help assess nutritional status
   b. To determine the degree of overnutrition or undernutrition
3. Interpretation of data
   a. IBW above 120% indicates obesity
   b. IBW below 90% may indicate undernutrition

**G. Body frame size**
1. General information
   a. Body frame size is classified as small, medium, or large
   b. Measurement requires a flexible, nonstretchable tape measure
   c. To determine body frame size, the examiner measures the circumference of the client's wrist at the smallest point, distal to the styloid process of the radius, then compares the measurement with reference standards for height by sex
   d. Body frame size is calculated by dividing the height (in cm) by the wrist circumference (in cm) and comparing to reference standards
2. Purposes
   a. To use in reference standards for determining IBW
   b. To use as a reference in height and weight tables that allow for differences in body frame size
3. Interpretation of data
   a. Small frame: greater than 10.4 cm (4″) for men; greater than 10.9 cm (4¼″) for women
   b. Medium frame: 9.6 to 10.4 cm (3¾″ to 4″) for men; 9.9 to 10.9 cm (4″ to 4¼″) for women
   c. Large frame: less than 9.6 cm (3¾″) for men; less than 9.9 cm (4″) for women

**H. Mid-arm circumference (MAC)**
1. General information (See *Anthropometric measurement standards* for further information on mid-arm circumference, skinfold thickness, and mid-arm muscle circumference.)
   a. Measurement requires a nonstretchable tape measure and a nonpermanent ink pen

## ANTHROPOMETRIC MEASUREMENT STANDARDS

**MALES: AGE 18 TO 74**

| Test | Mean | Percentile | | | | |
|------|------|------|------|------|------|------|
| | | 50th | 75th | 85th | 90th | 95th |
| TSF (mm) | 12.9 | 12.0 | 16.0 | 19.5 | 22.0 | 25.5 |
| MAC (cm) | 32.4 | 32.3 | 34.5 | 35.7 | 36.7 | 38.1 |
| MAMC (cm) | 28.3 | 28.5 | 29.5 | 29.6 | 29.8 | 30.1 |

**FEMALES: AGE 18 TO 74**

| Test | Mean | Percentile | | | | |
|------|------|------|------|------|------|------|
| | | 50th | 75th | 85th | 90th | 95th |
| TSF (mm) | 24.9 | 24.0 | 31.0 | 35.1 | 38.0 | 43.0 |
| MAC (cm) | 30.1 | 29.3 | 32.6 | 34.8 | 36.4 | 38.7 |
| MAMC (cm) | 22.3 | 21.8 | 22.9 | 23.8 | 24.5 | 25.2 |

Data from National Health Survey 1976-1980; DHHS publication No. (PHS) 87-1688.

    b.  To determine MAC, the examiner measures arm circumference halfway between the acromion process of the scapula and the tip of the elbow, records the measurement to the nearest millimeter, and compares it to reference standards for a normal arm measurement

2.  Purposes
    a.  To assess skeletal muscle mass, an important indicator of caloric intake
    b.  To use in the equation to determine mid-arm muscle circumference

3.  Interpretation of data: Measurement of less than 90% of the reference standard may indicate the need for nutritional support

## I.  Skinfold thickness

1.  General information
    a.  Approximately one-half of the body's fat stores lie directly beneath the skin in the subcutaneous layer
    b.  Common measurement sites include the triceps, subscapular area, suprailiac area, abdomen, and upper thigh
    c.  Triceps and subscapular measurements are the most useful because of the accurate reference standards that exist for them
    d.  Measurement requires a flexible, nonstretchable tape measure, a nonpermanent ink pen, and skinfold calipers

e. To determine skinfold thickness, the examiner picks up the skin and subcutaneous fat layer between the thumb and forefinger and measures it with a skinfold caliper to the nearest 0.5 mm. To compensate for any measurement error, the examiner should take three consecutive measurements and average the results

2. Purposes
   a. To measure subcutaneous fat stores, which reflect caloric reserves
   b. To use in determining mid-arm muscle circumference
3. Intrepretation of data
   a. Triceps skinfold (TSF) measurement of less than 90% of reference standard may indicate the need for nutritional support
   b. TSF greater than 15 mm in men and 25 mm in women indicates obesity

**J. Mid-arm muscle circumference (MAMC)**
1. General information
   a. Using the MAMC calculation, the examiner estimates the lean body mass of the arm, which correlates with body protein status
   b. Calculation of MAMC requires MAC and TSF measurements
   c. To calculate MAMC, the examiner uses the formula:
      MAMC (cm) = MAC (cm) − [3.14 × TSF (cm)]
2. Purposes
   a. To estimate body protein status
   b. To measure the amount of muscle or lean body mass
3. Interpretation of data: MAMC measurement of less than 90% of reference standards may indicate the need for nutritional support

**K. Diagnostic studies related to nutrition**
1. General information
   a. Various diagnostic studies help detect, rule out, or confirm certain nutritional deficiencies
   b. Diagnostic study results may indicate a marginal or subclinical nutritional deficiency before overt signs of malnutrition develop
   c. Results provide more objective assessment data than either clinical observation or a dietary history
2. Types of diagnostic studies
   a. Radiologic studies provide data about abnormally slow or rapid linear growth; used to assess growth and maturation problems and to detect such specific nutritional deficiencies as scurvy and rickets
   b. Organ function tests, such as respiratory function tests, are used in conjunction with measures of nutritional status to detect vital organ dysfunction, a possibly life-threatening effect of severe malnutrition
   c. Biochemical tests provide data on levels of certain nutrients and metabolites in body fluids or tissues; used to evaluate certain biochemical functions that depend on an adequate supply of essential nutrients, nutrient metabolism, and the body's response to nutritional interventions

**L.  Serum albumin**
  1.  General information
      a.  The most abundant plasma protein, serum albumin helps maintain plasma osmotic pressure and transport other nutrients and hormones through the blood
      b.  Serum albumin is formed in the liver, with synthesis depending on functioning liver cells and adequate supply of amino acids
      c.  Blood level tends to remain stable except in response to serious protein deficiency or loss of blood protein from burns, major surgery, infections, or cancer
      d.  Variables affecting test results include pregnancy, use of certain drugs, and high dietary fat intake before testing
  2.  Purpose in nutrition: To help assess visceral protein stores
  3.  Normal values
      a.  Adult: 3.5 to 5.0 g/dl
      b.  Child: same as adult
      c.  Newborn: 3.6 to 5.4 g/dl
  4.  Indications of abnormal values
      a.  Decreased levels: malnutrition, liver or renal disease, congestive heart failure, excessive blood protein losses such as from severe burns
      b.  Value of less than normal: specific indicator of protein-energy malnutrition in absence of other known causes

**M.  Serum transferrin**
  1.  General information
      a.  This transport protein regulates iron absorption and transport
      b.  Serum transferrin level, also called total iron binding capacity (TIBC), measures the quantity of transferrin by determining the amount of iron with which transferrin can bind
      c.  Serum transferrin level changes fairly rapidly in response to a change in body protein status
      d.  Variables affecting test results include iron status, pregnancy, age, and use of certain drugs
  2.  Purpose in nutrition: To help assess visceral protein stores; has a shorter half-life than serum albumin and thus more accurately reflects current status
  3.  Normal values
      a.  Adult: 250 to 410 mcg/dl
      b.  Child: 350 to 450 mcg/dl
      c.  Newborn: 60 to 175 mcg/dl
  4.  Indications of abnormal values
      a.  Increased TIBC: iron deficiency, as in pregnancy or iron-deficiency anemia
      b.  Decreased TIBC: iron excess, as in chronic inflammatory states
      c.  Below 200 mcg/dl: visceral protein stores depletion
      d.  Below 100 mcg/dl: severe visceral protein stores depletion

## N. Hemoglobin (Hgb)

1.  General information
    a.  The main component of red blood cells (RBCs), hemoglobin serves as a vehicle for transporting oxygen in the blood
    b.  Hemoglobin requires adequate protein for formation; is composed of amino acids that form *globin* and a red pigment portion called *heme*
    c.  Variables affecting test results include high altitudes, excessive fluid intake, infancy, pregnancy, and use of certain drugs
2.  Purposes in nutrition
    a.  To assess the oxygen-carrying capacity of blood
    b.  To help diagnose anemia, protein deficiency, and hydration status
3.  Normal values
    a.  Older adult: 10 to 17 g/dl
    b.  Adult male: 13 to 18 g/dl
    c.  Adult female: 12 to 16 g/dl
    d.  Child: 9.0 to 15.5 g/dl
    e.  Newborn: 14 to 20 g/dl
4.  Indications of abnormal values
    a.  Decreased values: protein deficiency, iron-deficiency anemia, excessive blood loss, overhydration
    b.  Increased values: dehydration, polycythemia

## O. Hematocrit (Hct)

1.  General information
    a.  This test determines the space occupied by packed RBCs; plasma and blood cells are separated by centrifugation
    b.  Test results are expressed as percentage of RBCs in a volume of whole blood
    d.  Variables affecting test results include high altitudes, pregnancy, age, and sex
2.  Purpose in nutrition: To help diagnose anemia and dehydration
3.  Normal values
    a.  Males: 42% to 50%
    b.  Females: 40% to 48%
4.  Indications of abnormal values
    a.  Decreased values: iron-deficiency anemia, excessive blood loss
    b.  Increased values: severe dehydration, polycythemia

## P. Total lymphocyte count (TLC)

1.  General information
    a.  This test measures white blood cells (WBCs) and, after calculation, lymphocytes
    b.  It is one means of evaluating immune system integrity; also provides information about the adequacy of visceral protein stores

  c.  WBCs, which fight infection, are formed in lymphatic tissues, including the spleen, thymus, and tonsils
  d.  TLC is calculated by multiplying the WBC count by the percentage of lymphocytes and dividing by 100
  e.  Variables affecting test results include hourly body rhythm, age, dietary intake, exercise, emotional stress, and use of certain drugs
2.  Purpose in nutrition: To help diagnose protein-energy malnutrition
3.  Normal values: 1,500 to 3,000 mm$^3$
4.  Indications of abnormal values
  a.  Decreased values: moderate to severe malnutrition if no other cause, such as influenza or measles, is identified
  b.  Increased values: infection or inflammation, leukemia, tissue necrosis

## Q.  Skin sensitivity testing
1.  General information
  a.  Also called antigen skin testing, this study helps evaluate immune system integrity and response by reflecting the status of cell-mediated immunity
  b.  This study involves placing small amounts of recall antigens under the skin and evaluating the resultant antibody synthesis and antibody response to stimulation
2.  Purpose in nutrition: To evaluate immune response, which is compromised in protein-energy malnutrition
3.  Normal results: Immunocompetent clients exhibit a positive reaction within 24 hours, marked by a red area of 5 mm or greater at the test site
4.  Indications of abnormal response: Delayed, partial, or negative reaction (no response) may point to protein-energy malnutrition

## R.  Creatinine-height index (CHI)
1.  General information
  a.  In this test, which helps evaluate protein metabolism, a 24-hour urinary creatinine value is compared with the standard value for the client's height
  b.  About 2% of creatine phosphate in muscle tissue is converted to creatinine each day; creatinine circulates in blood and is excreted in urine
  c.  Excretion rate depends on the amount of muscle mass: the more muscle mass, the greater the excretion; standard rates of excretion are determined from a reference table
  d.  Studies suggest that creatinine excretion decreases with age
  e.  This test has a high probability for error; it should not be used for clients with impaired renal function or in a catabolic state such as that associated with severe infections, trauma, or burns
  f.  High dietary protein intake may influence test results
2.  Purpose in nutrition: To determine the adequacy of muscle mass
3.  Normal values: Determined from a reference table for each client

    4. Indications of abnormal values
      a. Less than 80% of reference-standard value: moderate depletion of muscle mass (protein reserves)
      b. Less than 60% of reference-standard value: severe depletion, with increased risk of compromised immune function

**S. Fasting plasma glucose**
    1. General information
      a. Also known as fasting blood sugar (FBS), this test measures the plasma glucose level, which may reflect the adequacy of carbohydrate metabolism
      b. May be done by various techniques, such as venous sample or fingerstick
    2. Purpose in nutrition: To help evaluate carbohydrate metabolism
    3. Normal values: Generally between 60 and 100 mg/dl, but may vary according to laboratory procedure
    4. Indications of abnormal values
      a. 140 mg/dl or greater on two or more occasions: diabetes mellitus
      b. Less than 60 mg/dl: functional or reactive hypoglycemia

**T. Urine glucose**
    1. General information
      a. This test measures glucose levels in urine using a glucose reagent strip
      b. Glucosuria usually is present when blood glucose level exceeds 160 mg to 180 mg/dl, the usual renal threshold for glucose
    2. Purposes in nutrition
      a. To evaluate carbohydrate metabolism by detecting glucosuria
      b. To monitor glucose levels during insulin and total parenteral nutrition therapies
    3. Normal results: No glucose present in urine
    4. Indications of abnormal results: Hyperglycemia

**U. Total cholesterol**
    1. General information
      a. Cholesterol exists in muscles, RBCs, and cell membranes; is transported by low- and high-density lipoproteins; and is used by the body to form steroid hormones, bile acids, and cell membranes
      b. This test helps detect disorders of blood lipids
      c. Variables affecting test results include age, pregnancy, and use of estrogen and certain other drugs
    2. Purposes in nutrition
      a. To evaluate lipid metabolism
      b. To help assess dietary cholesterol intake
    3. Normal values
      a. Desirable range under scientific study
      b. Adult: 120 to 220 mg/dl

c.  Child: 135 to 250 mg/dl
d.  Infant: 70 to 190 mg/dl
4.  Indications of abnormal values
   a.  Less than 150 mg/dl: hypocholesterolemia
   b.  Greater than 220 mg/dl: hypercholesterolemia
   c.  Greater than 400 mg/dl: marked hypercholesterolemia

## V.  Triglycerides
1.  General information
   a.  Produced in the liver from glycerol and fatty acids, triglycerides are used in energy production
   b.  Excess amounts are stored in adipose tissue
   c.  This test provides an indication of the body's ability to metabolize fat
   d.  Variables affecting test results include alcohol ingestion, pregnancy, and oral contraceptive use
2.  Purposes in nutrition
   a.  To help detect protein-energy malnutrition
   b.  To screen for hyperlipidemia
3.  Normal values: 40 to 150 mg/dl
4.  Indications of abnormal values
   a.  Elevated levels in combination with elevated cholesterol levels: increased risk of atherosclerotic disease
   b.  Decreased levels: protein-energy malnutrition, steatorrhea

## W.  Urine ketone bodies (acetone)
1.  General information
   a.  Ketones are formed in the liver and completely metabolized in healthy persons
   b.  Ketone bodies in urine result from metabolism of fatty acids in states of carbohydrate deprivation, such as occurs in starvation or diabetic ketoacidosis
   c.  Ketone bodies in urine indicate that fat is the predominant source of body fuel
   d.  Variables affecting test results include use of carbohydrate-free diets, high-protein and high-fat diets, and certain drugs
2.  Purposes in nutrition
   a.  To screen for ketonuria
   b.  To detect carbohydrate deprivation
3.  Normal results: No ketone bodies in urine
4.  Indications of abnormal results: Ketoacidosis starvation

## Points to Remember

An initial nutritional screening, using nutritional assessment techniques, can help determine a client's nutritional status and identify steps necessary to maintain or help restore good nutritional status.

Steps of nutritional assessment include obtaining a nursing health history related to nutritional status, performing a physical assessment, reviewing pertinent laboratory test results and other records related to nutrition, consulting with other health team members such as dietitians, and reviewing current literature related to nutritional care.

To prevent errors in obtaining and interpreting anthropometric data, the examiner should use standard equipment and procedures and appropriate standards for each index used.

Diagnostic study results may indicate a marginal or subclinical nutritional deficiency before overt signs of malnutrition develop.

## Glossary

**Anthropometry**—science of body measurements

**Polycythemia**—abnormal increase in the erythrocyte count or in hemoglobin concentration

**Standard**—established measurement or model for comparative studies

**Steatorrhea**—excessive fat in feces, as occurs in malabsorption syndrome

# Standard Hospital Diets

**Learning Objectives**

After studying this section, the reader should be able to:

- Describe the uses of hospital diet manuals.

- Describe the purpose of a progressive dietary regimen.

- Compare and contrast the characteristics of clear liquid, full liquid, soft, and regular diets.

- List the indications for using standard hospital diets.

- Identify foods allowed in each standard hospital diet.

- Describe the nursing implications associated with using clear liquid, full liquid, soft, and regular diets.

## XXI. Standard Hospital Diets

### A. Introduction

1. Almost every health care institution has prepared or adopted a diet manual compiled of routine, modified, or test diets used in that institution
2. Such diet manuals serve the following purposes:
   a. Provide guidelines for physicians ordering diets
   b. Act as tools to enhance communication among health team members concerned with clients' nutritional status
   c. Provide rationales for specific diets, lists of foods allowed and prohibited in each diet, sample menus, and nutritional evaluations
   d. Serve as teaching tools and reference documents for nurses, physicians, and other health care professionals
3. The most commonly used diets in hospitals include:
   a. Regular diets
   b. Diets modified in texture, including liquid (clear and full liquid) and soft diets; also known as progressive hospital diets
4. A progressive dietary regimen provides nutritional support as the client progresses from a clear liquid to full liquid to soft to regular diet

### B. Clear liquid diet

1. General information
   a. Intended for short-term use, usually no longer than 24 to 48 hours
   b. Highly restrictive, composed of foods that are transparent and liquid or that liquefy at room temperature
   c. Involves fluid restriction of 30 to 60 ml/hr, gradually increased to match client tolerence
   d. Provides an inadequate daily nutritional intake: contains 600 to 900 calories; 5 to 15 grams of protein, primarily from gelatin (an incomplete protein); no fat; and 100 to 130 grams of carbohydrates
2. Indications
   a. Difficulty chewing or swallowing
   b. Temporary food intolerance resulting from nausea, vomiting, abdominal distention, or diarrhea
   c. Preoperatively or postoperatively to maintain electrolyte balance
   d. Before certain diagnostic tests to reduce colonic fecal matter content
3. Foods allowed
   a. Water, ice chips
   b. Tea
   c. Decaffeinated coffee; inclusion in clear liquid diet may vary with institutional policy
   d. Fruit juices (strained and clear)
   e. Carbonated beverages (clear)
   f. Plain gelatin
   g. Broth (fat-free only)

    h. Bouillon
    i. Frozen ice pops (clear)
    j. Fruit-flavored drink mixes (clear)
  4. Nursing implications
    a. Explain the rationale for this diet to the client and family
    b. Assess the client's tolerence of the diet
    c. Auscultate for bowel sounds
    d. Monitor intake and output
    e. Discuss with the physician any improvement in the client's status that indicates he can be advanced to full liquid diet

## C. Full liquid diet
  1. General information
    a. Used as a transition diet between a clear liquid diet and a soft diet, usually short-term
    b. Includes foods that are liquid at room temperature and foods that liquefy at body temperature
    c. May provide adequate nutrition with careful planning, except for fiber and iron content
    d. Provides 2,000 calories, 70 grams of protein, 80 grams of fat, and 250 grams of carbohydrates daily
    e. Contraindicated for clients with severe lactose intolerance and, unless modified, for long-term use in clients with hypercholesterolemia
  2. Indications
    a. Postoperatively
    b. Acute infections and fever of short duration
    c. Lack of appetite
    d. Intolerance of solid foods, as with GI disturbances
    e. Difficulty chewing and swallowing
  3. Foods allowed
    a. All liquids on clear liquid diet
    b. All forms of milk
    c. Soup, including strained vegetable, meat, or cream
    d. Fruit and vegetable juices
    e. Cooked and strained cereals
    f. Soft custards
    g. Plain ice cream, sherbets
    h. Puddings
  4. Nursing implications
    a. Explain to the client and his family the rationale for this diet
    b. Recommend modifications to increase calories and protein if the diet is used longer than 2 to 3 days
    c. Provide lactose-reduced milk for a client with lactose intolerance
    d. Adapt the diet as appropriate for a client with diabetes mellitus, renal disease, or other disorders

e. Use low-sodium products for a client requiring sodium restriction
f. Assess the client for changes in status, such as increased appetite and changed bowel sounds
g. Discuss with the physician any improvement in the client's status that indicates he can be advanced to a soft diet

## D.  Soft diet
1. General information
   a. Used as a transition diet between a full liquid diet and a regular diet
   b. Modified in texture using foods low in fiber, connective tissue, and fat
   c. Provides adequate nutrition; planned to meet the recommended dietary allowance (RDA) for calories and nutrients
   d. Available in two forms: regular (or traditional) soft and mechanical soft
2. Indications
   a. Postoperatively
   b. Convalescence from acute infections
   c. Mild GI disturbances
   d. Chewing difficulties resulting from lack of teeth, ill-fitting dentures, or oral surgery
3. Foods allowed
   a. All liquids included in the full liquid diet
   b. Bananas (ripe)
   c. Breads and cereals (refined)
   d. Cakes and cookies (plain)
   e. Cheese (cottage, American, and mild cheddar)
   f. Eggs
   g. Fats (oils, mayonnaise, French dressing)
   h. Fruits (cooked, without skins or seeds)
   i. Meat (ground and tender)
   j. Pasta (noodles, macaroni, spaghetti)
   k. White rice
   l. Vegetables (low-fiber, cooked without skins)
4. Nursing implications
   a. Explain to the client and his family the rationale for this diet
   b. Help the client make menu choices according to his food preferences
   c. Teach the client and family about foods allowed on the diet and appropriate preparation methods
   d. Assess the client for changes in status
   e. Discuss with the physician any improvement in the client's status that indicates he can be advanced to a regular diet

## F.  Regular diet
1. General information
   a. Also known as a normal, general, or house diet
   b. Is the most commonly used standard hospital diet

    c. Uses a normal, healthy person as a standard for nutrient requirements

    d. Contains all essential nutrients for the client's age and sex and meets RDA requirements

2. Indications

    a. Intended to maintain health

    b. Used for clients requiring no particular modifications in diet

3. Foods allowed

    a. No foods excluded, except for personal dislikes

    b. No restrictions on portion size

4. Nursing implications

    a. Encourage the client to choose a variety of foods from the four basic food groups

    b. Monitor the client's nutritional status during hospitalization to ensure adequate nutrient intake

## Points to Remember

A client's diet should be advanced to the next step as soon as possible.

A progressive dietary regimen provides nutritional support as the client progresses from a clear liquid diet to a regular diet.

The clear liquid diet provides inadequate levels of all nutrients and should be used short-term only.

A full liquid diet includes foods that are liquid at room temperature or liquefy at body temperature.

## Glossary

**Hypercholesterolemia**—excessive serum cholesterol level

**Lactose intolerance**—inablility to tolerate milk or milk products because of deficiency of the enzyme lactase, which breaks down lactose (milk sugar)

**Mechanical soft diet**—foods that can be eaten without chewing; used for clients who have difficulty chewing

# Special Hospital Diets

**Learning Objectives**

After studying this section, the reader should be able to:

- Describe various vegetarian diets.

- Describe the important dietary practices related to the Jewish faith.

- Describe the important dietary practices related to the Islamic faith.

## XXII. Special Hospital Diets

### A. Introduction
1. Special diets are based on religious laws or perceived health values
2. Various religions, such as Judaism and Islam, specify dietary restrictions and practices based on religious laws
3. Standard hospital diets may violate a client's religious dietary laws or personal dietary practices
4. Knowledge of a client's special dietary needs is necessary to ensure healthful nutrition while also respecting the client's beliefs and preferences

### B. Vegetarian diets
1. General information
   a. Vegetarianism is increasing in the United States, particularly among young adults; about 7 million Americans consider themselves vegetarians
   b. People become vegetarians for religious, health, ethical-ecological, or economic reasons
   c. Various religions—including Seventh-day Adventists and certain Eastern religious sects—advocate vegetarianism
   d. Vegetarian diets generally require more time for meal planning and preparation than do traditional diets
   e. Vegetarians often have difficulty obtaining a well-balanced vegetarian diet when away from home
2. Types of vegetarian diets
   a. Vegetarianism involves eating plant-derived foods only
   b. Lacto-vegetarianism allows adding dairy products to a diet of plant foods
   c. Lacto-ovo-vegetarianism allows adding dairy products and eggs to a diet of plant foods
   d. Fruitarianism limits the diet to fresh raw fruits, juices, and nuts and seeds
3. Food sources
   a. Grains, legumes, nuts, and seeds: six servings or more daily, including several slices of yeast-raised whole-grain bread, a serving of beans, and a few nuts or seeds
   b. Vegetables: three or more servings daily, including one or more servings of dark leafy greens
   c. Fruit: one to four pieces daily, including a raw source of vitamin C
   d. Milk and eggs: two or more glasses of fresh milk per day for adults, three or more per day for children (other dairy products or an egg may be used to meet part of the daily milk requirement); eggs optional, up to four per week
4. Nursing implications
   a. Advise the client to gather information about essential and nonessential amino acids and to incorporate it into his diet; many authorities feel vegetarians don't get the necessary essential amino acids

  b.  Advise the client to avoid foods that provide few nutrients and empty calories
  c.  Inform the client that according to some authorities four to six servings of complementary proteins should be eaten daily to ensure adequate intake of essential amino acids
  d.  Advise the client to eat more whole grain breads and cereals and milk products to meet caloric requirements
  e.  Encourage the client to eat a variety of foods to ensure adequate quantity and quality of protein intake
  f.  Advise the client to include a rich source of vitamin C at every meal to enhance iron absorption
  g.  Advise the client who is following veganism to eat foods high in iron, calcium, and zinc and that he will need vitamin $B_{12}$ supplements
  h.  Recommend that the client eat foods that contain adequate amounts of other required nutrients or, if this is not possible, advise him to take nutrient supplements

**C.  Religious dietary laws: Judaism**
  1.  General information
    a.  Jews traditionally have used food in religious feasts and ceremonies
    b.  Jewish dietary laws are based on Biblical and rabbinical regulations
    c.  Diet is regulated by a body of laws known as the *rules of kashruth,* which define foods that are kosher, or fit
    d.  The rules of kashruth specify that all meats must be kosher, and that meats and dairy products cannot be served together
    e.  Specific dietary practices vary among Jews, according to their particular group affiliation and country of origin
  2.  Types
    a.  Orthodox Jews strictly observe the traditional dietary laws at all times
    b.  Conservative Jews adhere nominally to the dietary laws and sometimes make a distinction between observing them inside and outside the home
    c.  Reformed Jews may minimize the significance of the dietary laws, regarding them as mainly ceremonial
  3.  Food sources
    a.  Kosher meats
    b.  Fish with fins or scales
    c.  Eggs
    d.  All fruits and vegetables
    e.  All grain products
    f.  Milk and dairy products—but not with meat
  4.  Prohibited foods
    a.  All products obtained from pigs, including pork, bacon, and animal shortening
    b.  Shellfish, eels, and scavenger fish

      c. Non-kosher meat
      d. Meat and poultry in combination with dairy products
   5. Nursing implications
      a. Suggest that a client on a tight budget use less expensive cuts of meat or other sources of protein, such as fish and cheese (when in accordance with dietary laws), rather than more expensive kosher meats
      b. Discourage excessive use of delicatessen-type meats, such as corned beef and pastrami, because of their high sodium and fat content
      c. Encourage the consumption of various vegetables, including green leafy and yellow ones
      d. Suggest the use of fruit juices rather than soft drinks as a beverage for meat-based meals
      e. Allow adequate time for hygiene rituals before meals

**E. Religious dietary laws: Islam**
   1. General information
      a. Islamic dietary laws are similar to Jewish kosher laws
      b. The various Islamic groups interpret the dietary laws in different ways
      c. Slaughtering of animals for meat must be done in the name of Allah following a specific ritual
   2. Food sources
      a. Meats slaughtered in accordance with the prescribed ritual
      b. Fish, shellfish, and poultry
      c. Honey and dates
      d. Sweets
      e. Vegetable oils
      f. Fruits, vegetables, and grains
      g. Milk and dairy products
   3. Prohibited foods
      a. Pork, animal shortening, and gelatin
      b. Other products from animals not slaughtered in accordance with the prescribed ritual
      c. Alcoholic beverages and alcohol-containing products, including flavoring extracts
      d. Stimulating beverages, including coffee and tea
   4. Nursing implications
      a. Keep in mind the prohibited foods when adapting special diets; make appropriate substitutions
      b. Allow the client adequate time for hygiene rituals before meals

## Points to Remember

Special diets are based on religious dietary laws or perceived health values.

Various religions, such as Judaism and Islam, specify dietary restrictions and practices based on religious laws.

A standard hospital diet may violate a client's religious dietary laws or personal dietary practices.

Knowledge of a client's special dietary needs is necessary to ensure healthful nutrition while also respecting the client's beliefs and preferences.

## Glossary

**Complementary proteins**—protein formed when foods deficient in certain essential amino acids but adequate in others are combined in the diet to ensure adequate intake of essential amino acids

**Kosher**—process that removes blood from meat and poultry before cooking; involves soaking the flesh in water, salting it, draining it, and then washing it 3 times to remove the salt

**Vegetarianism**—practice of restricting the diet to vegetables, fruits, grains, and nuts; may include milk, milk products, and eggs; excludes all animal flesh

# Therapeutic Diets

**Learning Objectives**

After studying this section, the reader should be able to:

• Explain the use of the nursing process in providing therapeutic nutrition.

• Describe the purpose of selected therapeutic diets.

• Discuss selected therapeutic diets, including foods allowed and not allowed.

• List important nursing implications associated with selected therapeutic diets.

## XXIII. Therapeutic Diets

### A. Introduction

1. Therapeutic diets involve modifications of nutritional components necessitated by a client's disease state or nutritional status
2. Therapeutic diets modify specific nutrients or types of food
3. Therapeutic nutrition is an important part of treatment, even when it is not emphasized
4. Therapeutic diets have proven effective—and sometimes vital—in treating various disorders, including diabetes mellitus, celiac disease, and lactose intolerance
5. Providing therapeutic nutrition involves:
   a. *Assessing* the client's mental, emotional, and physical status (including status of the client's GI tract); the appropriateness of the prescribed therapeutic diet to the client's altered health or nutritional status; and the client's ability to understand the diet and comply with it
   b. *Planning* and analyzing the prescribed therapeutic diet to match the client's nutritional requirements, tolerance, and compliance
   c. *Implementing* the prescribed therapeutic diet and appropriate client teaching
   d. *Evaluating* the client's response to the therapeutic diet
6. Dietary restrictions in therapeutic diets range from conservative to rigid
7. A client must know or be taught the importance of adhering to his prescribed therapeutic diet, even when he feels better and thinks he no longer needs it

### B. Calorie-modified diet: Decreased

1. General information
   a. This diet is designed to promote weight loss while providing adequate nutrition
   b. Recommended rate of weight loss is 1 to 2 lb per week
   c. Caloric intake for overweight and mildly obese clients usually ranges from 1,000 to 1,200 calories per day for women and 1,200 to 1,500 calories per day for men
   d. This diet may not promote adequate weight loss in some moderately or morbidly obese clients. Such clients may find a very-low-calorie diet (VLCD), also known as a protein-sparing modified fast (PSMF) diet, more effective
2. Indications
   a. Overweight
   b. Mild obesity
   c. Moderate obesity
   d. Morbid obesity
3. Foods allowed
   a. Fresh fruits and vegetables prepared without added fat
   b. Lean meats, poultry without skin, fish

      c.  Breads, pasta, rice, potatoes, dried peas and beans, corn, fresh peas, winter squash, unsweetened cereals
      d.  Whole grain and high-fiber foods
      e.  Skim milk and low-fat dairy products
      f.  Herbs and spices
  4.  Foods not allowed
      a.  Fried foods
      b.  Sweetened cereals
      c.  High-fat foods, such as butter, bacon, shortening, ice cream
      d.  Desserts laden with sugar, such as Danish, donuts, cookies, candy
      e.  Whole milk dairy products, such as ice cream, sour cream, certain cheeses
  5.  Nursing implications
      a.  Explain the rationale for the decreased-calorie diet
      b.  Enlist the support of the client's family in encouraging client compliance
      c.  Suggest that the client plan shopping lists and menus to avoid impulse buying and eating
      d.  Encourage the client to eat three meals a day and to eat fresh fruit and vegetables for between-meal snacks to avoid extreme hunger, which may lead to binge eating
      e.  Encourage the client not to abandon the diet if he "cheats"; explain that occasional noncompliance usually won't affect his long-term success
      f.  Teach the client about using behavior modification techniques to improve compliance

**C.  Fiber-modified diet: Increased**
  1.  General information
      a.  This is essentially a normal diet that substitutes high-fiber foods for low-fiber foods
      b.  It includes at least four servings of fruits and vegetables per day, preferably fresh and raw
      c.  Because fiber isn't completely digestible, this diet increases mechanical stimulation of the GI tract
      d.  Objectives of this diet include increasing fecal bulk, increasing GI motility, and decreasing pressure within the bowel
  2.  Indications
      a.  Constipation
      b.  Diverticulosis
      c.  Irritable bowel syndrome
      d.  Diabetes, to improve glucose tolerance
      e.  Hypercholesterolemia, to help lower serum cholesterol levels
  3.  Food sources
      a.  Whole grain breads and cereals, especially products made with bran
      b.  Vegetables: raw or cooked with minimum preparation, especially carrots, peas, broccoli, corn, lettuce, dried peas and beans

    c. Fresh fruits with the skin on (especially apples and pears), berries, oranges, and stewed and dried fruits

    d. Nuts and seeds

  4. Nursing implications

    a. Explain the rationale for the high-fiber diet

    b. Initiate the diet slowly to develop client tolerance

    c. If symptoms of intolerance appear—such as flatus, distention, cramping, and diarrhea—reduce the fiber content to the maximum amount tolerated by the client

    d. Monitor laboratory study results for signs of calcium, zinc, or iron deficiency; these minerals may be eliminated in feces because of the increased intestinal transit time

    e. Encourage intake of foods rich in calcium, zinc, and iron to help prevent deficiencies

    f. If deficiencies develop, provide calcium, zinc, or iron supplements as appropriate

    g. Teach the client minor changes in eating and cooking habits that can help increase his fiber intake

    h. Explain that certain high-fiber foods, such as prunes and prune juice, figs, and dates, also have laxative effects

    i. Encourage the client to drink at least six to eight 8-oz glasses of water daily while on the high-fiber diet

**D. Fiber-modified diet: Decreased**

  1. General information

    a. This diet, also known as a low-residue diet, restricts dietary fiber and residue to eliminate or reduce mechanical stimulation of the GI tract

    b. Dietary restrictions vary considerably among clients and institutions and range from mild to severe

    c. Objectives of this diet include reducing stool bulk and slowing transit time through the bowel

  2. Indications

    a. Bowel inflammation, as seen in the acute stages of diverticulosis, ulcerative colitis, and regional enteritis

    b. Esophageal and intestinal stenosis

    c. Preparation for bowel surgery

  3. Foods allowed

    a. Meat: ground or well-cooked tender meat, fish, poultry

    b. Eggs

    c. Dairy products: up to 2 cups of milk per day, mild cheese

    d. Fruits: strained fruit juices, except prune; cooked or canned apples, apricots, white cherries, peaches, pears, ripe bananas

    e. Vegetables: strained vegetable juice; canned, cooked, or strained asparagus, beets, green beans, pumpkin, acorn squash, spinach

    f.  Breads and cereals: white bread, toast, crackers, bagels, Melba toast, waffles, and refined cereals such as Cream of Wheat, Cream of Rice, and puffed rice

    g.  Miscellaneous: plain desserts made with allowed foods; gelatin; candy such as butterscotch, jellybeans, marshmallows, and plain hard candy; honey, molasses, and sugar

4.  Foods not allowed

    a.  Meats: tough meats

    b.  Dairy products: more than 2 cups of milk per day

    c.  Fruits: all raw, cooked, or dried fruits not listed

    d.  Vegetables: all raw or cooked vegetables not listed

    e.  Breads and cereals: whole grain breads and cereals, especially those made with bran or cracked wheat

    f.  Miscellaneous: nuts, peanut butter, coconut, and anything made with nuts or coconut; olives and pickles; seeds

5.  Nursing implications

    a.  Explain to the client the rationale for the low-fiber diet and that reducing fiber intake will slow the passage of food through the bowel

    b.  Teach the client that fiber is a component of plants and therefore is found in fruits, vegetables, and grains

    c.  Explain to the client that milk and milk products are limited because they leave a residue after digestion

    d.  Explain to the client that skins, seeds, and membranes of fruits and vegetables are high in fiber and should be removed

    e.  Teach the client to cook allowed vegetables until very tender

    f.  Monitor laboratory study results and observe for signs of calcium deficiency resulting from restrictions on intake of milk and dairy products

    g.  Monitor laboratory study results and observe for signs of iron deficiency resulting from such factors as the client's refusal to eat ground meat (a rich source of iron) and restriction of other sources of iron, such as dried fruits and iron-fortified cereals

    h.  Monitor laboratory study results and observe for signs of vitamin deficiency resulting from restrictions on vegetable intake and processing techniques of allowed vegetables that remove vitamins as well as fiber

    i.  Encourage the client to eat as varied a diet as possible within the restrictions, and advance the diet as soon as possible

    j.  Monitor for inadequate caloric intake, especially important because of the diet's restrictions

    k.  Assess for constipation related to the diet's low fiber content, which causes a decrease in stool bulk and slows intestinal transit time

    l.  Eliminate all fruits and vegetables except for strained fruit juice if persistent diarrhea occurs from poor tolerance of even small amounts of fiber

**E. Protein-modified diet: Increased**
   1. General information
      a. Protein requirements increase when caloric intake is inadequate or marginal, when protein intake is of poor quality and doesn't supply all of the essential amino acids, and during healing and other hypermetabolic states
      b. Objectives of this diet include meeting increased protein requirements needed for tissue repair and while combatting infection, and replacing the lean body mass lost during the catabolic phase following extreme physiologic stress
   2. Indications
      a. Hypermetabolic conditions, such as burns, sepsis, and major trauma
      b. Protein-energy malnutrition
      c. Cancer cachexia
      d. Major surgery
      e. Peritoneal dialysis
      f. Multiple fractures
      g. Protein-wasting renal diseases, such as nephrotic syndrome
      h. Hepatitis
      i. Malabsorption syndromes, including protein-wasting enteropathy, short-bowel syndrome, inflammatory bowel diseases, and celiac disease
   3. Food sources
      a. Milk: contains complete protein
      b. Meat: contains complete protein
      c. Vegetables: contain incomplete protein
      d. Bread and cereals: contain incomplete protein
   4. Nursing implications
      a. Explain to the client the rationale for increasing his dietary protein intake
      b. Teach the client about food sources of protein
      c. Monitor serum albumin, iron, and transferrin levels and total lymphocyte count, and observe for signs of protein-energy malnutrition
      d. Monitor anthropometric measurements for changes indicating muscle wasting
      e. Monitor dietary protein intake and calculate the requirements approved for the client's nutritional status

**F. Protein-modified diet: Decreased**
   1. General information
      a. The degree of protein restriction depends on the client's laboratory study data and clinical symptoms
      b. The client's protein intake is adjusted and modified to promote nitrogen balance while maintaining blood urea nitrogen (BUN) levels below 60 to 90 mg/dl
      c. This diet's main objective is to maintain or restore optimum nutritional status in clients with impaired ability to eliminate protein

2. Indications
   a. Anuric phase of acute renal failure (ARF)
   b. Chronic renal failure (CRF) not treated with dialysis
   c. Cirrhosis of the liver with signs of impending coma
3. Foods allowed
   a. Beverages: carbonated soft drinks, fruit drinks and punches, lemonade, limeade
   b. Candies: candy corn, fondant (candy made with egg white only), hard candies, gum, gumdrops, jelly beans, lollipops, marshmallows, mints
   c. Desserts: fruit ices, popsicles
   d. Fats: butter and margarine (unsalted), mayonnaise (no eggs), oils, shortening
   e. Flour products: arrowroot, cornstarch, rice starch, tapioca, wheat starch
   f. Sweeteners: corn syrup, honey, jams, jellies, maple syrup, confectioners' sugar
   g. Protein-free seasonings: flavoring extracts, herbs, spices, vinegar
   h. Fruits and vegetables: most varieties are allowed (depends on protein content and severity of restriction)
4. Foods not allowed: Foods high in protein, such as meats and dairy products
5. Nursing implications
   a. Explain the rationale for the low-protein diet
   b. Provide thorough diet teaching, and periodically evaluate the client's understanding
   c. Stress to the client the importance of viewing this diet as a vital part of his therapy
   d. Instruct the client to weigh himself daily, and to report any significant change
   e. Provide the client with the titles of appropriate cookbooks, particularly vegetarian cookbooks
   f. Encourage the client to take vitamin and mineral supplements as ordered by the physician
   g. Stress the importance of consistant, controlled protein intake; adequate caloric intake; fluid restrictions, if needed; and sodium restrictions, if appropriate
   h. Monitor intake and output to prevent fluid imbalances
   i. Observe for signs of nutritional excesses and deficiencies
   j. When calculating proper protein intake for clients with CRF, keep in mind the need for nitrogen balance; be aware of the narrow margin of safety in avoiding uremic toxicity (from excessive protein intake) while preventing malnutrition (from inadequate protein intake)
   k. As ordered, provide special commercial formulas containing essential amino acids as a dietary supplement

## G. Protein-modified diet: Low phenylalanine

1. General information
   a. Phenylalanine is an essential amino acid necessary for optimal growth
   b. Some infants are born with a congenital absence of phenylalanine hydroxylase, an enzyme that acts in metabolism of phenylalanine. This disorder, known as phenylketonuria (PKU), leads to accumulation of phenylalanine and its metabolic products, which can cause irreversible cerebral damage and mental retardation
   c. Although this diet may be difficult to follow, strict compliance is necessary to prevent complications of PKU
   d. The main objective is to reduce phenylalanine intake while providing sufficient amino acids and nutrients for normal growth and development
2. Indications: PKU
3. Foods allowed
   a. vegetables
   b. fruits
   c. some cereals, breads, and other starches only in measured amounts
4. Foods not allowed
   a. meat
   b. fish
   c. poultry
   d. milk and dairy products
   e. eggs
5. Nursing implications
   a. Explain the rationale for this special diet to the parents of a child with PKU
   b. Provide a diet adequate in protein-sparing calories to prevent the use of protein for energy, which can result in body protein catabolism
   c. Be aware that some researchers have recommended that children with PKU follow this diet to adolescence or even adulthood
   d. Provide formulas specially prepared for infants with PKU, such as Lofenelac (Mead), which has 95% of the phenylalanine removed
   e. Provide parents of infants ready for solid foods with meal patterns and exchange lists of foods grouped according to their phenylalanine content to aid diet planning
   f. Provide comprehensive and frequent diet counseling to assess the child's nutritional intake and progress
   g. Explain that the diet is low in phenylalanine, not phenylalanine-free, and must provide adequate calories
   h. Instruct the parents to read the labels on all packaged food to determine its phenylalanine content
   i. Instruct the parents not to give the child anything containing aspartame (Nutrasweet), which contains phenylalanine
   j. Advise the parents to explain the diet to the child as soon as he's able to understand it, and to encourage the child to become involved in dietary planning at an early age

## H. Protein-modified diet: Gluten-free
1. General information
   a. Gluten is a protein found in wheat and other grains that gives dough its elastic property
   b. Some infants and children have a disorder (celiac disease) that results in damage to the intestinal lining from the glutamine-bound fraction of protein
   c. The main objective is to provide adequate nutrients, prevent futher damage, improve symptoms, and correct nutrient malabsorption
2. Indications: celiac disease
3. Foods allowed
   a. Beverages: carbonated drinks, cocoa, coffee, tea, fruit juice, milk, decaffeinated coffee containing no wheat
   b. Breads and cereals: products made only with arrowroot, cornstarch, cornmeal, potato, rice, soybean, buckwheat, or gluten-free wheat starch flours; pure rice, sago, and tapioca; gluten-free macaroni products; cornbread, muffins, and pone made without wheat flour; corn and rice cereals, such as cornflakes and puffed rice
   c. Desserts: cakes, cookies, pastries, and other baked products made with allowed flours; custard; gelatin; cornstarch, rice pudding, tapioca pudding, ice cream, and sherbet prepared without gluten stabilizers
   d. Fats: butter, corn oil, french dressing, mayonnaise, olive oil, margarine, and other animal and vegetable fats and oils that contain no wheat or grain additions
   e. Soups: broth, bouillon, clear soups, cream soups thickened with allowed flours
   f. Miscellaneous: pepper, pickles, popcorn, potato chips, sugars and syrups, vinegar, molasses
4. Foods not allowed
   a. Beverages: ale and beer; instant coffee containing wheat; Postum, Ovaltine, and other cereal beverages; malted milk
   b. Breads and cereals: all products made from wheat, rye, oats, or barley, such as all commercial yeast and quick bread mixes, bran, crackers, macaroni, noodles, pancakes, pretzels, vermicelli, Zwieback; cooked or ready-to-eat cereals containing malt, bran, rye, wheat, oats, barley, or wheat germ
   c. Desserts: cakes, cookies, pastries, and other baked products made with restricted flours; prepared mixes and puddings thickened with wheat flour
   d. Fats: commercial salad dressings that contain gluten stabilizers, homemade salad dressings thickened with flour
   e. Miscellaneous: soups thickened with wheat products or containing barley, noodles, or other wheat, rye, or oat products in any form
5. Nursing implications
   a. Explain to the parents of a child on a gluten-free diet that all sources of gluten must be eliminated from the diet, and specify the foods to avoid

    b. Explain that the diet does not cure the disease but can relieve the symptoms after several weeks

    c. Instruct the parents to use substitute bread and flour products made from gluten-free wheat starch, potato, buckwheat, soybean, lima bean, arrowroot, cornmeal, or rice flour

    d. Point out the need to avoid foods that contain breading, gravy, cream sauces, or other restricted foods when eating away from home

    e. Stress that the client must follow the diet for life, as no cure yet exists for celiac disease

    f. Recommend ongoing follow-up with continuing dietary advice and counseling

    g. Recommend contacting the American Celiac Society and other groups that serve as valuable sources of dietary assistance

    h. Provide the parents with names of manufacturers of gluten-free food products

## I. Protein-modified diet: Low purine

  1. General information

    a. Purines exist in nucleoproteins that are in all foods and most abundant in high-protein foods

    b. Uric acid is the metabolic end product of purines

    c. Because the body synthesizes purines, diet modifications alone can't control a high uric acid level

    d. The main objective is to restrict the amount of purines to lower serum uric acid levels while supplying adequate nutrients

  2. Indications

    a. Gout

    b. Renal calculi

    c. Increased uric acid levels secondary to obesity, hypertension, hypertriglyceridemia, alcoholism, lead toxicity, pregnancy-induced hypertension, leukemia, polycythemia, psoriasis, or diuretic therapy

  3. Foods allowed:

    a. Any food containing less than 150 mg of purines per 100 g

    b. Limited amounts of foods containing moderate amounts of purines, such as meats and dairy products

  4. Foods not allowed

    a. Organ meats: liver, kidney, sweetbreads, brains, heart

    b. Fish: mussels, anchovies, sardines, fish roe, herring, shrimp, mackerel

    c. Meat extracts: meat drippings, gravy broth, consommé

    d. Miscellaneous: mincemeat, yeast

  5. Nursing implications

    a. Recommend that the client drink at least 2 quarts of water and fruit juice daily to decrease the risk of renal calculi formation and to prevent the dehydration associated with anti-gout medications

    b. Encourage the client to maintain a low-fat diet; explain that a high-fat diet can increase the frequency of acute gout attacks

c. Recommend a diet limiting protein to 50 to 75 g/day, with most of it from plant and dairy sources
d. Discourage consumption of alcoholic beverages, which can aggravate gout
e. Discourage fasting, low carbohydrate diets, and rapid weight loss; all favor the formation of ketones, which inhibit the excretion of uric acid
f. Encourage a high carbohydrate diet, which generally tends to increase uric acid excretion; however, discourage high fructose (fruit sugar) intake, which may increase uric acid production
g. Encourage a high intake of fruits and vegetables to increase urine alkalinity and thereby increase the solubility of uric acid
h. Explain that avoidance of coffee, tea, and cocoa is no longer considered necessary

**J. Protein-modified diet: Tyramine-free**
1. General information
    a. Tyramine, a vasoactive amine found in some protein food sources, affects the GI tract and central nervous system by stimulating the release of epinephrine and norepinephrine
    b. Monoamine oxidase (MAO) inhibitors alter the body's metabolism of tyramine, causing an elevated tyramine level
    c. Eating foods containing tyramine while taking MAO inhibitors produces strong pressor responses, such as hypertension and occipital headache, from adding to the already elevated tyramine levels
    d. The main objective is to supply adequate nutrients while restricting tyramine to prevent nutrient and drug interactions
2. Indications: MAO inhibitor therapy
3. Foods allowed: Any food that does not contain tyramine
4. Foods not allowed
    a. Dairy products: sharp or aged cheese such as blue, Boursault, brick, Brie, Camembert, cheddar, Emmenthaler, Gruyère, mozzarella, Parmesan, Romano, Roquefort, and Stilton; sour cream; yogurt
    b. Meats and fish: fermented meat, fish, poultry, and sausage; caviar; chicken liver; pickled herring
    c. Fruits and vegetables: broad beans, avocados, bananas, canned figs, raisins
    d. Beverages: beer, Chianti, other wines in large quantities, sherry
5. Nursing implications
    a. Explain the rationale for avoiding foods containing tyramine
    b. Explain that hypertensive crisis may occur following the ingestion of MAO inhibitors with foods containing tyramine
    c. Teach the client the signs and symptoms of hypertensive crisis, such as severe headache, blurred vision, nausea, or vomiting, and the need to inform the physician immediately if any occur

## K.  Sodium-modified diet: Decreased

1.  General information
    a.  This diet can involve varying degrees of sodium restriction: mild, moderate, strict, and severe
    b.  Lists that specify the sodium content of foods may provide greater dietary flexibility
    c.  Restrictions are based on the total daily sodium intake, not on specific intake of certain foods
    d.  This diet is contraindicated in clients with sodium-wasting renal disease, such as pyelonephritis, polycystic renal disease, and bilateral hydronephrosis; pregnancy; clients with ileostomies; and myxedema
    e.  Clients on strict or severe sodium restriction usually are hospitalized and have an unusually low sodium tolerance
    f.  In some areas, drinking water may naturally contain significant sodium levels; in hard-water areas, sodium-based water softeners may elevate sodium levels
    g.  Variable amounts of sodium may be ingested through such medications as barbiturates, sulfonamides, antibiotics, cough medicines, laxatives, and antacids
    h.  The objective of this diet is to limit sodium intake because sodium promotes fluid accumulation associated with certain disorders
2.  Indications
    a.  Liver disease characterized by edema and ascites
    b.  Treatment and possible prevention of hypertension
    c.  Congestive heart failure
    d.  Renal disease characterized by edema and hypertension
    e.  Adrenocortical therapy
3.  Foods allowed
    a.  Mild sodium restriction (2,000 mg to 3,000 mg): food may be lightly salted during cooking
    b.  Moderate sodium restriction (1,000 mg to 2,000 mg): allow either ¼ teaspoonful of salt in cooking or at the table and use unsalted bread and butter, or use no salt in cooking or at the table but allow measured amounts of regular bread and butter; low-sodium products are allowed
    c.  Strict sodium restriction (500 mg): foods low in sodium
    d.  Severe sodium restriction (250 mg): same restrictions apply as for strict sodium restriction with addition of low-sodium milk only and limited amounts of meats and eggs
4.  Foods not allowed
    a.  Mild sodium restriction (2,000 mg to 3,000 mg): no salt may be added to food at the table; foods high in added sodium are prohibited
    b.  Moderate sodium restriction (1,000 mg to 2,000 mg): foods high in added sodium are prohibited
    c.  Strict sodium restriction (500 mg): no salt may be added to food at the table or used in cooking; foods high in added sodium and naturally high in sodium are prohibited

      d. Severe sodium restriction (250 mg): same restrictions apply as for strict sodium restriction

5. Nursing implications

      a. Explain to the client how the low-sodium diet will help to control his disease

      b. Explain that sodium is present, either naturally or by addition, in many foods providing other essential nutrients

      c. Assure the client that the taste for salt decreases with time, making compliance with sodium restrictions easier

      d. Suggest the use of other seasonings, such as herbs and spices, to increase the palatability of food

      e. Explain changes in meal planning, shopping, food preparation, and in eating out necessitated by sodium restriction

      f. Help the client set realistic goals for diet modification that relate to his economic, cultural, and social situation

      g. Instruct the client to rinse the contents of canned foods under running water for at least 1 minute to remove most of the added sodium

      h. Explain that the sodium-containing compounds that add the largest amounts of sodium to foods are table salt, baking soda (sodium bicarbonate), monosodium glutamate (MSG), baking powder, and brine

      i. Instruct the client to examine food labels for other sodium compounds often added as preservatives or flavor enhancers, such as sodium benzoate, sodium citrate, sodium propionate, sodium alginate, sodium sulfite, sodium hydroxide, disodium phosphate, and sodium saccharin

      j. Inform the client that many over-the-counter medications—notably antacids and cold medicines—contain high sodium levels; instruct him to read the labels

      k. Instruct the client to thoroughly rinse his mouth after brushing or using mouthwash to prevent absorption of the sodium contained in toothpaste and mouthwash

      l. Encourage the client's family to show support by also following the diet, if possible

      m. Provide reading materials—such as those available from the American Heart Association—that describe sodium-restricted diets

      n. Provide the titles of various low-sodium cookbooks

      o. Recommend consulting with a dietitian-nutritionist for suggestions on altering recipes to comply with sodium restrictions

      p. Monitor for signs and symptoms of hyponatremia (such as nausea, malaise, possible confusion, seizures, and coma) related to a low sodium intake with concomitant use of diuretics, particularly in elderly clients or those with renal disease

      q. Initiate a low-sodium diet gradually in clients with renal disease and elderly clients to allow their homeostatic mechanisms time to adapt

**L.  Fat-modified diet: Decreased**
  1.  General information
      a.  This diet limits total daily fat intake to approximately 30 to 50 g, regardless of type
      b.  It specifies that foods be baked, broiled, or boiled instead of fried or prepared with added fat
      c.  Visible fat on meats must be trimmed and poultry skin removed, preferably before cooking
      d.  Allowed fats can be used as seasonings or in cooking
      e.  Fat exchanges may be used in menu planning
      f.  The objective of this diet is to reduce symptoms of steatorrhea and pain in clients intolerant of fat
  2.  Indications
      a.  Chronic pancreatitis
      b.  Malabsorption syndromes
      c.  Some cases of gallbladder disease
      d.  Hyperlipidemia
  3.  Foods allowed
      a.  Meats: up to 6 oz of lean meat, fish, and skinless poultry daily; up to three egg yolks per week; egg whites and low-fat egg substitutes as desired
      b.  Dairy products: skim milk; skim milk cheeses, yogurt, and pudding
      c.  Fruits and vegetables: any prepared without added fat, except avocados
      d.  Bread and cereals: plain cereals, pasta, macaroni, rice, whole grain or enriched breads
      e.  Miscellaneous: sherbet, fruit ices, gelatin, angel food cake, fat-free or skim milk soups, soft drinks, honey, sugar, seasonings as desired
      f.  Fats: up to six servings daily of polyunsaturated vegetable oils; corn, cottonseed, safflower, sesame, or soybean oil; margarines and liquid oil shortenings
  4.  Foods not allowed
      a.  Meats: fatty meats, sausage, lunch meat, spare ribs, frankfurters, salt pork, tuna and salmon packed in oil
      b.  Dairy products: whole milk, whole milk cheeses and yogurt, ice cream
      c.  Fruits and vegetables: any buttered, au gratin, creamed, or fried vegetables
      d.  Breads and cereals: products made with added fat, such as biscuits, muffins, pancakes, doughnuts, waffles, and sweet rolls; breads made with eggs, cheese, or added fat
      e.  Miscellaneous: gravy; peanut butter; desserts, candy, and any food containing chocolate or nuts
  5.  Nursing implications
      a.  Encourage the client to eat a variety of allowed foods
      b.  Instruct the client to reduce or eliminate fat exchanges and limit the amount of low-fat meat allowed if symptoms of steatorrhea persist or if pain occurs after eating

    c. Monitor laboratory study results and observe for signs of iron deficiency from limited allowance of meat, especially red meats

    d. Suggest iron supplements, if needed

    e. Encourage increased intake of low-fat, high-iron foods, such as dried fruits, fortified cereals and grains, green leafy vegetables, and dried peas and beans

    f. Instruct the client to eat a reliable source of vitamin C at each meal to enhance iron absorption from plant sources

    g. Instruct the client that the goal is to reduce the total amount of fat ingested, regardless of the source

    h. Teach the client strategies for complying with his diet when dining out

    i. Teach the client food preparation techniques that help reduce fat content

    j. Advise the client to purchase lean cuts of meat and avoid marbled fat that cannot be trimmed off

## M. Cholesterol and triglyceride-modified diet: Decreased

  1. General information

    a. The American Heart Association (AHA) recommends that all people follow a diet low in cholesterol, triglycerides, and saturated fats

    b. The objective of this diet is to reduce the risk of developing cardiovascular disease by reducing serum lipid levels

    c. This diet also usually specifies an increase in dietary fiber, which reduces the serum cholesterol level, and in unsaturated fat

    d. The AHA has recommended three levels of cholesterol and triglyceride restriction, from slightly restrictive to severely restrictive

  2. Indications

    a. Atherosclerotic heart disease

    b. Hypertension

    c. Obesity

    d. Diabetes mellitus

    e. Gout

    f. Hyperlipidemia

    g. To reduce the risk of cardiovascular disease

  3. Foods allowed

    a. Vegetable oils, such as safflower, sunflower, soybean, sesame, corn, cottonseed, linseed, peanut; mayonnaise and salad dressing made with these oils

    b. Margarines: soft and semisolid

    c. Chicken: breast and thigh without skin

    d. Freshwater fish

    e. Walnuts and almonds

    f. Oat bran and oatmeal (high-fiber)

    g. Dried peas and beans (high-fiber)

    h. Peas, corn, sweet potatoes, zucchini, cauliflower, broccoli, prunes, pears, apples, bananas, oranges (high-fiber)

4. Foods not allowed
   a. Excessive calories from any source that promotes or maintains obesity
   b. Foods high in saturated fat: coconut and palm oils; butter and lard; beef, pork, veal, and mutton; chicken liver; egg yolk; whole milk and whole milk products
   c. Foods high in cholesterol: organ meats such as liver, heart, sweetbreads, brains, and kidney; shrimp and sardines; egg yolk; meat; shellfish such as crabs, clams, lobster, oysters, and scallops; whole milk and whole milk products; ice cream and ice milk
5. Nursing implications
   a. Explain the rationale for the diet to the client and his family
   b. Explain that saturated fats, found mainly in animal products, tend to raise serum cholesterol; monounsaturated and polyunsaturated fats, found mainly in plant foods, tend to lower serum cholesterol levels
   c. Suggest instituting dietary changes gradually
   d. Encourage the intake of fruit, soybeans, oats, and oat products, which are known to lower serum cholesterol levels
   e. Advise the client to follow the AHA's dietary guidelines
   f. Refer the client to the local AHA chapter for additional resources
   g. Instruct the client on food preparation techniques to reduce saturated fat content
   h. Teach the client how to read food product labels to identify sources of saturated fats
   i. Provide the client with appropriate teaching materials related to diet

**N. Carbohydrate-modified diet: Decreased**
1. General information
   a. This diet—often called a diabetic diet—is used mainly in clients with diabetes mellitus, an endocrine disorder resulting from faulty carbohydrate metabolism and characterized by an elevated blood glucose level related to insulin deficiency
   b. The diabetic diet most commonly used is the one recommended by the American Diabetes Association (ADA), adapted to individual caloric requirements and based on food group exchange lists
   c. Often, a diabetic client does not require a decrease in total daily carbohydrate intake, but a reallocation of carbohydrate intake throughout the day to control blood glucose levels
   d. In diabetic clients, the objective of diet therapy is to maintain blood glucose levels as near as possible to normal
2. Indications
   a. Diabetes mellitus
   b. Weight reduction
3. Foods allowed
   a. With the exception of pure sugar and foods high in sugar, most foods can be calculated into the food exchanges

      b.  Carbohydrates: emphasis on grains, vegetables, and legumes

      c.  Fats: limited saturated fats and cholesterol; slight increase in polyunsaturated fats

      d.  Protein: emphasis on sources low in fat and low in saturated fat and cholesterol

      e.  Sodium: in moderation

  4.  Foods not allowed

      a.  Dairy products: chocolate and condensed milk, milkshakes, ice cream, puddings

      b.  Fruits and vegetables: any fruit or vegetable canned, frozen, or cooked with sugar; sweetened fruit drinks, ices, and juices; cranberry sauce; glazed vegetables

      c.  Breads and cereals: sweet rolls, coffee cakes, sweetened cereals

      d.  Miscellaneous: cakes, candy, chewing gum, cookies, doughnuts, sweetened gelatin, honey, jam and jelly, marmalade, molasses, pastries, pies, popsicles, soft drinks, sherbet, sugar, and syrup

  5.  Nursing implications

      a.  Explain the rationale for the diabetic diet to the client and his family

      b.  Provide the client with appropriate exchange lists and explain how to use them correctly

      c.  Encourage the client to eat the prescribed amount of food at each meal and snack and never to skip meals and snacks

      d.  Advise the diabetic client to always carry a source of rapidly absorbed sugar, such as hard candy, in the event of an unexpectedly delayed meal or drop in blood sugar

      e.  Advise the client to be aware of a decrease in appetite that may lead to inadequate food intake and result in hypoglycemia

      f.  Advise the client to monitor his weight carefully and to inform his physician of any significant weight loss

      g.  Advise the client to eat extra carbohydrates before engaging in moderate or vigorous exercise to prevent hypoglycemia

      h.  Explain that medication may be used in addition to diet therapy, but not as a substitite for diet

      i.  Provide the client with food preparation ideas

      j.  Teach the client how to order from a menu when dining out

      k.  Advise the client on food purchasing and label reading

      l.  Provide the client with diabetic recipes and titles of diabetic cookbooks

      m.  Advise the client about the resources provided by the ADA

**O.  Lactose-modified diet: Decreased**

  1.  General information

      a.  This diet limits lactose (milk sugar) for clients with lactose intolerance caused by deficiency of the digestive enzyme lactase

      b.  Lactose is the main form of carbohydrate in milk and dairy products

      c.  Lactose intolerance occurs most commonly in Blacks, Orientals, Jews, and Native Americans; affects only 6% to 8% of Whites

2. Indications: Primary (congenital), secondary, or acquired lactose intolerance
3. Foods allowed: Any food that does not contain lactose
4. Foods not allowed
   a. Milk: whole, 2%, 1%, skimmed, evaporated, nonfat dry milk, milk solids
   b. Cream and sour cream
   c. All cheese, except aged natural cheeses
   d. Cream soups and sauces
   e. Specialty-flavored instant coffee blends made with dairy creamers
   f. Cocoa and most chocolate beverages
   g. Ice cream, custard, pudding
5. Nursing implications
   a. Explain the rationale for the diet to the client and his family
   b. Observe for symptoms of lactose intolerance, such as abdominal distention and cramps, flatus, and diarrhea, occurring 15 to 30 minutes after ingestion of milk and other dairy products
   c. Be aware that tolerance to lactose varies widely among affected clients and that diet restrictions may not be permanent; reduce lactose only to the maximun amount tolerated by the client
   d. Monitor for signs and symptoms of calcium deficiency and provide supplements as needed
   e. Encourage increased intake of nondairy foods high in calcium, such as green leafy vegetables, carrots, dates, prunes, canned sardines and salmon with bones, oranges, egg yolks, whole grains, nuts, and dried peas and beans, to prevent calcium deficiency from reduced milk intake
   f. Instruct the client to read food labels carefully to identify sources of lactose
   g. Inform the client that he may tolerate acidophilus milk or lactose-reduced milk
   h. Explain that lactose-free nondairy creamer can be used in beverages, on cereal, and in cooking, if desired

**P. Iron-modified diet: Increased**
1. General information
   a. Iron comes in two forms: *heme iron,* which constitutes about half of the iron found in such animal sources as meat, fish, and poultry; and *nonheme iron,* which constitutes the remaining half of the iron found in animal sources and all of the iron found in plant sources, such as grains, vegetables, legumes, and nuts
   b. Nonheme iron accounts for the greater percentage of total dietary iron intake
   c. Relatively few foods provide excellent sources of dietary iron
   d. On average, only 10% of the iron consumed is absorbed
   e. Iron deficiency anemia is the most common nutritional deficiency disorder in the United States

2. Indications
   a. Increased dietary iron requirements related to accelerated growth in pregnancy, infancy, or puberty
   b. Heavy or chronic blood loss, such as with menstruation, surgery, injury, childbirth, or GI bleeding
   c. Decreased iron absorption related to the use of certain medications
   d. Iron deficiency anemia
   e. Inadequate dietary iron intake, as may occur, for example, in persons of low income and in vegetarians
   f. Inadequate iron absorption, as may occur from chronic diarrhea or malabsorption syndrome
3. Foods allowed
   a. Sources of *heme iron:* beef (muscle meats, heart, kidney, liver, and tongue), chicken and turkey (especially dark meat), pork loin and sausage, lamb, veal, egg yolk, clams, oysters, sardines, shrimp
   b. Sources of *nonheme iron:* bran flakes; oatmeal; brewer's yeast; brown rice; chocolate and cocoa; enriched and whole grain breads, cereals, and flours; fortified cereals; dried beans, peas, soybeans, and lentils; sweet potatoes; dried fruit (apricots, currants, dates, figs, peaches, prunes, raisins); greens (beet, dandelion, kale, spinach, Swiss chard, turnip); molasses; nuts (almonds, Brazil nuts, cashews, hazelnuts, pecans, peanuts, walnuts)
4. Foods not allowed
   a. Tea
   b. Coffee
5. Nursing implications
   a. Advise the client to eat foods containing heme iron at every meal
   b. Advise the client to consume a rich source of vitamin C at every meal to enhance absorption of nonheme iron
   c. Tell the client to avoid foods known to inhibit nonheme iron absorption
   d. Advise the client to cook in iron pots whenever possible
   e. Recommend that the client take iron supplements, as appropriate
   f. Monitor serum iron, TIBC, and Hgb to evaluate results of therapy

Q. **Calcium-modified diet: Increased**
   1. General information
      a. Calcium is the body's most abundant mineral, constituting about half of the total mineral content
      b. Bones constantly take up and release calcium to maintain serum calcium levels within a narrow normal range
      c. Only 10% to 30% of dietary calcium is absorbed; the remaining 70% to 90% is excreted in urine and feces
      d. Calcium deficiency may be related to inadequate calcium intake or may occur secondary to malabsorption syndrome, vitamin D deficiency, or endocrine disorders

2. Indications
   a. Osteoporosis
   b. Osteomalacia
   c. Alveolar bone loss
   d. Hypertension
   e. Malabsorption syndrome
   f. Hypoparathyroidism
3. Food sources
   a. Dairy products
   b. Canned fish with bones, such as pink salmon and sardines
   c. Green leafy vegetables, such as collards, kale, and turnip greens
   d. Organ meats
   e. Refined carbohydrates rather than high-fiber carbohydrates
4. Nursing implications
   a. Be aware that dietary fiber can bind with calcium, decreasing the amount of calcium available for absorption
   b. Teach the client that maintaining a diet rich in calcium, phosphorus, and vitamin D through adolescence and early adulthood helps ensure proper bone formation and peak bone mass entering late adulthood
   c. Explain that even in adulthood, a person needs a diet rich in calcium to help minimize bone loss
   d. Point out that some evidence suggests that elderly persons, especially women, need a higher calcium intake than that specified in the recommended dietary allowance (RDA) charts
   e. Teach the client that vitamin D is essential to the absorption and conservation of calcium
   f. Advise the client to avoid smoking, excessive intake of caffeine, protein, fiber, and alcohol to help prevent interference with calcium absorption or use
   g. Advise a client with lactose intolerance to use low-lactose milk or to use enzyme preparations available to reduce the lactose content of milk
   h. Advise the client to use calcium supplements, as appropriate

**R. Calcium-modified diet: Decreased**
   1. General information
      a. An excessive serum calcium level results in hypercalciuria, which can lead to precipitation and calculi formation
      b. Hypercalciuria may be related to excessive dietary calcium, sugar, and animal protein intake or may occur secondary to endocrine disorders, bone disorders, or prolonged immobility
   2. Indications
      a. Renal calculi
      b. Bone disease
      c. Hyperparathyroidism
      d. Prolonged immobility

3. Foods allowed
   a. Nondairy, noncarbonated drinks
   b. Yellow vegetables
   c. Whole-grain breads and other carbohydrate sources, such as pasta and unprocessed bran
4. Foods not allowed
   a. Carbonated soft drinks
   b. Dairy products
   c. Cocoa, peanuts, spinach and other leafy green vegetables
   d. Organ meats and other animal sources of protein
   e. Refined foods, such as cakes and cookies
5. Nursing implications
   a. Explain the rationale for this diet to the client and his family
   b. Stress the importance of following the prescribed dietary and medication regimen
   c. Instruct the client to include dietary fiber at each meal to help speed intestinal transit time and increase calcium binding, which will decrease calcium absorption
   d. Encourage a client with renal calculi to increase fluid intake

## Points to Remember

Therapeutic diets have proven effective in treating various disorders; in some cases, diet therapy plays a vital role in a client's physical recovery.

Therapeutic diets that focus on limiting sodium, cholesterol, and fat intake play a major role in preventing cardiovascular disease.

The nurse's role in client-teaching about therapeutic diets includes assessing the client's understanding of and ability to comply with the dietary regimen, providing any further information (with the assistance of the dietitian) as needed, and stressing the importance of compliance.

## Glossary

**Alveolar bone**—bone that forms the socket of a tooth

**Diverticulosis**—blind pouch formed from the mucous membrane of the intestine

**Gout**—metabolic disease marked by urate deposits in joints that result in painful arthritis; linked to a genetic defect in purine metabolism

**Hypercalciuria**—excessive calcium in urine

**Hypercholesterolemia**—excessive cholesterol in the blood

**Phenylketonuria (PKU)**—congenital disease resulting from an inborn error of metabolism of the amino acid phenylalanine

# Enteral Nutrition

**Learning Objectives**

After studying this section, the reader should be able to:

• Discuss the general characteristics of enteral nutrition.

• Describe the types of formulas used in enteral nutrition.

• List the indications for using enteral nutrition.

• Describe the different routes for administering enteral nutrition.

• Discuss nursing implications associated with enteral nutrition.

## XXIV. Enteral Nutrition

### A. Introduction

1. Enteral nutrition is a convenient and economical method of nutritional support when oral feeding is not adequate or feasible
2. Except when using monomeric formulas, the client on enteral nutrition must have a functioning GI tract
3. Enteral nutrition can be used as the sole feeding method or as a supplement to oral feeding
4. Enteral nutrition is available in various formulas to meet different nutritional needs; these formulas differ in osmolarity, digestibility, caloric density, lactose content, viscosity, and fat content
5. Advantages of enteral nutrition
   a. Maintains GI tract integrity with food digestion and nutrient absorption
   b. Requires minimal digestion before nutrient absorption can take place
   c. Costs less than parenteral nutrition; specifically, in the formula, the equipment, and staff time
   d. Is much safer than parenteral nutrition, with decreased risk of infection, fluid and electrolyte imbalance, and complications of catheterization

### B. Types of formulas

1. *Blended tube feedings* consist of normal foods blended to a liquid consistency, such as Compleat B (Doyle) and Formula 2 (Cutter). Used for clients with a functioning GI tract but with oral or swallowing problems
2. *Polymeric formulas* provide complete nutrient intake in a complex form. May be milk-based, such as Meritene (Doyle) and Instant Breakfast (Carnation), or lactose-free, such as Ensure (Ross), Isocal (Mead-Johnson), and Osmolite (Ross). Use requires a normally functioning GI tract
3. *Monomeric formulas* are elemental or chemically defined diets. These hypertonic formulas usually are supplied in powder form to be mixed with water; examples include Criticare (Mead-Johnson) and Vivonex (Eaton). Use does not require a functioning GI tract
4. *Modular feeding components* are individual nutrients designed to increase dietary intake of proteins, carbohydrates, or fats. Products include Polycose (Ross), MCT Oil (Mead-Johnson), and Casec (Mead-Johnson)
5. *Specialty feedings* are special formulations designed for particular metabolic problems. Products include Amin-aid (McGaw) and Travasorb (Travenol). Use requires a functioning GI tract

### C. Indications

1. Physical impairments
   a. Swallowing difficulties
   b. Dental disorders
   c. Dysphagia
   d. Stroke complications, such as paralysis

2. GI tract problems
   a. Esophageal fistula
   b. Partial obstructions in the esophagus or pylorus
   c. Surgery or radiation therapy of the upper alimentary tract, neck, upper respiratory system, or oropharynx
   d. Inflammatory bowel diseases, such as Crohn's disease
   e. Colitis
   f. Malabsorption syndrome
   g. Enterocutaneous fistulas
   h. Pancreatic insufficiency
   i. Short-bowel syndrome
   j. Partial bowel obstruction
3. Psychological disturbances
   a. Depression
   b. Anorexia nervosa
   c. Bulimia
4. Hypermetabolic states
   a. Burns
   b. Sepsis
   c. Multiple trauma
   d. Cancer
   e. Hyperthyroidism
5. Alterations in consciousness
   a. Coma
   b. Delirium
   c. Dementia

**D. Routes of administration**
1. General information
   a. Enteral nutrition is administered through tubes made of soft, nonirritating polyurethane or silicon with radiopaque mercury or tungsten weights at the base
   b. Tubes may be inserted nonsurgically through the nose or mouth or surgically through an opening into the GI tract
2. Intragastric tubes are preferred for short-term feedings. Types of intragastric tubes include:
   a. Nasogastric (NG) tubes, which are passed through the nose into the stomach
   b. Orogastric tubes, which are passed through the mouth into the stomach
   c. Nasoduodenal (ND) tubes, which are passed through the nose into the duodenum
   d. Nasojejunal (NJ) tubes, which are passed through the nose into the jejunum

3.  Ostomy tubes are more suitable for long-term use. Types of ostomy tubes include:
    a.  Esophagostomy tubes, which are inserted surgically into one of several esophageal sites (cervical or thoracic) and advanced into the stomach
    b.  Gastrostomy tubes, which are inserted surgically through the skin of the abdomen and into the stomach
    c.  Jejunostomy tubes, which are inserted surgically through the skin of the abdomen and into the jejunum

E.  **Methods of delivery**
    1.  General information
        a.  Small, dilute feedings are administered initially
        b.  Volume and concentration are gradually increased as tolerated by the client
    2.  Bolus feedings
        a.  Bolus feedings are delivered to the stomach only
        b.  They normally are administered every 3 to 4 hours to resemble a normal meal pattern
        c.  Approximately 100 to 400 ml are administered at each feeding, using an Asepto syringe or slow gravity drip
        d.  Clients usually better tolerate the prescribed volume of formula when it's infused over 20 to 30 minutes using a slow gravity drip
    3.  Continuous feedings
        a.  Continuous feedings are administered by gravity drip or volumetric pump through a tube with a lumen smaller than No. 8 French. The pump is more dependable because of its constant flow rate
        b.  Continuous feedings usually are administered over 16 to 24 hours
        c.  Continuous feedings improve absorption, reduce diarrhea, and achieve nitrogen balance more rapidly than bolus feedings
        d.  A continuous infusion pump is recommended for feedings into the distal duodenum or proximal jejunum, for delivering monomeric formulas, and for feeding clients with limited absorptive capability

F.  **Nursing implications for enteral nutrition**
    1.  Check the diet and fluid order before administering any tube feedings
    2.  Check the formula for expiration date, time that it was opened, and the time it has been kept at room temperature
    3.  Before administering the feeding, determine tube position and patency and the amount of gastric residue present
    4.  To help prevent aspiration, position the client sitting upright or with the head of the bed elevated 30 to 45 degrees, if possible
    5.  When administering a bolus feeding, notify the physician if you obtain 100 ml or more of aspirate, and replace any aspirate to prevent loss of gastric juices and electrolytes
    6.  When feeding through an NG tube, use the smallest caliber tube feasible and provide frequent nasal care to decrease irritation to the nares

7. When feeding through any intragastric tube, provide oral hygiene—unless contraindicated by oral surgery

8. If the client complains of cramping or nausea, slow the rate or reduce the concentration of the feeding

9. If the client vomits, stop the feeding immediately to prevent aspiration

10. Increase the client's water intake if constipation occurs because of low residue in feedings

11. Do not allow feedings to remain at room temperature for more than 6 to 8 hours; the formulas provide excellent media for bacteria growth

12. Do not add new formula to a feeding than has been hanging for more than 6 hours

13. Add any prescribed medications at the beginning of a bolus feeding. Use liquid or powdered forms of drugs if possible; crushed tablets may clog the tube

14. Administer antidiarrheal drugs such as diphenoxylate hydrochloride with atropine sulfate (Lomotil) or paregoric for persistent diarrhea, as ordered

15. Flush the tube with at least 30 ml of water before and after administering any medication

16. Add pectin, applesauce, or mashed banana to the feeding to help thicken stools, if necessary and feasible

17. Encourage the client to walk whenever possible—or provide physical therapy for a bedridden client—to prevent constipation, increase use of proteins that occurs during activity, and improve morale

18. When adminstering low-fat formulas that do not contain the essential fatty acids, monitor for fatty acid deficiency, which is characterized by dry, itchy skin

## Points to Remember

Enteral nutrition is a convenient and economical method of nutritional support when oral feeding is not adequate or feasible.

Except when using monomeric formulas, the client on enteral nutrition must have a functioning GI tract.

Enteral nutrition can be used as the sole feeding method or as a supplement to oral feeding.

Enteral nutrition is available in various formulas to meet different nutritional needs; these formulas differ in osmolarity, digestibility, caloric density, lactose content, viscosity, and fat content.

Intragastric tube feedings are best for short-term feeding; ostomy tube feedings are more suitable for long-term use.

## Glossary

**Aspiration**—act of breathing or drawing vomitus or food into the respiratory tract

**Bolus**—concentrated mass of food or liquid introduced to the GI tract

**Monomeric formula**—preparation of hydrolyzed nutrients that is ready to be absorbed and requires no digestive secretions

**Polymeric formula**—preparation that provides intact nutrients requiring a normally functioning GI tract for absorption

# Parenteral Nutrition

## Learning Objectives

After studying this section, the reader should be able to:

• List the nutrients that can be supplied parenterally.

• Compare and contrast the use of peripheral veins and central veins for administering parenteral solutions.

• Explain the general characteristics of total parenteral nutrition (TPN).

• List the purposes and indications for using TPN.

• Describe the nursing implications associated with TPN.

# XXV. Parenteral Nutrition

## A. Introduction

1. Parenteral nutrition is delivered intravenously through a peripheral or central vein
2. Parenteral nutrition provides adequate nutritional intake when enteral nutrition is insufficient or contraindicated
3. The usual fluid volume administered to an adult is 3 liters over 24 hours
4. The specific composition of parenteral solutions depends on the client's nutrient requirements and health status

## B. Parenteral nutrients

1. General information
   a. Parenteral nutrition can supply all the basic required nutrients: protein, carbohydrates, lipids, vitamins, and minerals
   b. The addition of alcohol provides an additional source of energy (7 calories per gram of alcohol)
2. Energy (calories)
   a. In parenteral nutrition, caloric intake is usually calculated by the solution's carbohydrate content (unless fats or alcohol are included)
   b. Parenteral nutrition provides 3.4 calories per gram of carbohydrate
   c. The body uses calories supplied parenterally less efficiently than those given enterally
3. Carbohydrates
   a. Parenteral nutrition supplies carbohydrates in the form of monosaccharides, such as dextrose, fructose, and invert sugar
   b. Insulin may be necessary during administration of hypertonic dextrose solutions to prevent hyperglycemia and glucosuria
4. Protein
   a. Administration of protein solution is recommended when parenteral fluids are given for more than 3 to 4 days
   b. Protein solution provided in parenteral nutrition consists of crystalline compounds that contain both essential and nonessential amino acids
   c. These protein solutions are well tolerated and enhance protein synthesis and improve nitrogen balance when given in adequate amounts; they are expensive, however
   d. One liter of 5% amino acid solution provides 6.2 grams of nitrogen and 175 calories
5. Lipids
   a. In parenteral nutrition, lipids are supplied as fat emulsions
   b. Fat emulsions provide more than twice the energy of protein or carbohydrate solutions

    c. They are protein-sparing and comparable to glucose in promoting positive nitrogen balance

    d. They can be used with carbohydrate and amino acid solutions in both peripheral and central venous administration

    e. Fat emulsions provide 1.1 calories/ml with a 10% solution and 2 calories/ml with a 20% solution

    f. Available solutions include Intralipid (Cutter), a soybean oil emulsion, and Liposyn (Abbott), a safflower oil emulsion

    g. Administration of fat emulsions is necessary in long-term (longer than 3 weeks) total parenteral nutrition (TPN), to prevent essential fatty acid deficiency

    h. Administration should be initiated slowly and increased only as tolerated by the client

6. Vitamins

    a. Vitamin requirements for clients on long-term TPN have not been established

    b. A client receiving parenteral nutrition excretes greater-than-normal amounts of vitamins in urine

    c. A client receiving parenteral nutrition may require supplements of certain vitamins, such as folic acid, K, and $B_{12}$

7. Minerals

    a. Administration of mineral supplements is necessary for clients receiving long-term TPN

    b. Sodium requirements in parenteral nutrition range from 40 to 150 mEq/day

    c. Potassium requirements range from 70 to 150 mEq/day

    d. Chloride requirements equal sodium requirements

    e. Calcium requirements range from 0.2 to 0.3 mEq/kg/day

    f. Magnesium requirements range from 0.35 to 0.45 mEq/kg/day

    g. Phosphorus requirements vary widely, but generally range from 7 to 10 mmol/1,000 calories

    h. Serum levels of electrolytes and trace elements must be monitored closely during long-term TPN. Copper, molybdenum, iodine, selenium, or zinc supplements also may be necessary

## C. Peripheral parenteral nutrition (PPN)

1. General information

    a. PPN is considered a safer method for supplying nutrients than TPN through a central vein

    b. PPN may be used as an adjunct to oral or enteral feedings to provide adequate intake

    c. The variety of solutions is limited for use with PPN

    d.  The amount of nutrients provided to a client through PPN depends on the amount of infused fluid the client can handle safely

    e.  PPN usually is contraindicated for nutritionally depleted clients or clients with greatly increased nutritional needs because of hypermetabolic states

2.  Purposes

    a.  To maintain or restore fluid and electrolyte balance

    b.  To prevent deterioration and achieve homeostasis

    c.  To provide minimum caloric and protein requirements

3.  Indications

    a.  Preoperatively and postoperatively

    b.  Low-calorie support

    c.  Supplementation of enteral therapy when necessary

4.  Nutrient solutions

    a.  *5% dextrose in water (D₅W):* partially spares protein; nearly isotonic; inexpensive

    b.  *10% dextrose in water (D₁₀W):* provides more calories than D₅W; hyperosmolar; inexpensive

    c.  *Amino acid solution:* provides nitrogen to help achieve nitrogen balance; few adverse physiologic effects; nearly isotonic; hyperosmolar; expensive

    d.  *Protein hydrolysates:* lower in cost than synthetic amino acids; may precipitate an allergic reaction

    e.  *Fat emulsions:* used to prevent or correct essential fatty acid deficiency and to provide additional concentrated source of calories; isotonic; available in 10% to 20% concentrations

5.  Nursing implications for administering PPN

    a.  Check the physician's order to ensure the correct type and amount of solution to administer and the proper infusion rate

    b.  Explain the rationale for PPN and the procedure to the client and his family, if appropriate

    c.  Follow proper procedures for initiating I.V. therapy

    d.  Use sterile technique for procedures to prevent bacterial invasion of the circulatory system

    e.  Assess and monitor the client for clinical signs of fluid and electrolyte imbalance, such as fluid overload

    f.  Monitor intake and output

    g.  Remember that although solutions containing carbohydrates and water can be useful in preventing dehydration, they do not provide sufficient calories to maintain health or to promote wound healing, weight gain, or normal growth in children

**D.  Total parental nutrition (TPN)**

1.  General information

    a.  TPN, also called intravenous hyperalimentation (IVH) or simply hyperalimentation, consists of I.V. solutions of amino acids, glucose, fat emulsions, electrolytes, and other micronutrients

b. It usually is administered through an indwelling catheter inserted into a large central vein because of the need for rapid dilution of the hyperosmotic solutions
  c. TPN can be used to meet nutritional needs for a prolonged period and may be useful as a preventive therapeutic measure
  d. It can provide the calories required for tissue maintenance, usually in the range of 1,800 to 3,000/day
  e. TPN is the most complex and expensive method available for providing nutrients

2. Purposes
  a. To maintain or increase body weight
  b. To achieve normal growth or catch-up growth in infants and children
  c. To restore lean body mass and adipose tissue in wasted clients

3. Indications
  a. Debilitating illness lasting longer than 2 weeks
  b. Limited or no oral intake for longer than 7 days, as may occur in multiple trauma, severe burns, or anorexia nervosa
  c. Loss of 10% or more of baseline pre-illness weight
  d. Serum albumin level below 3.5 g/dl
  e. Poor tolerance of long-term enteral feedings
  f. Chronic vomiting or diarrhea
  g. Continued weight loss despite adequate oral intake
  h. GI disorders that prevent or severely reduce absorption, such as bowel obstruction, Crohn's disease, ulcerative colitis, short bowel syndrome, cancer, malabsorption syndrome, and bowel fistulas
  i. Inflammatory GI disorders, such as pancreatitis and peritonitis

4. Nutrient solutions
  a. *Admixtures of dextrose in water* (20% to 50%) and *crystalline amino acids*: other vitamins and minerals are added based on the client's laboratory data; hyperosmotic; expensive; provides total nutrients
  b. *Fat emulsions* (10% or 20%): prevent or correct essential fatty acid deficiency and provide additional calories; isotonic
  c. *Total nutritional admixtures (TNA)*: lipids premixed with dextrose and crystalline amino acids; provide all essential nutrients, including fats, in a convenient form; expensive; hyperosmotic

5. Nursing implications for administering TPN
  a. Check the physician's order to ensure the correct type and amount of solution to administer, the correct solution delivery system, and the proper infusion rate
  b. Explain the rationale for TPN and the procedure to the client and his family, if appropriate
  c. Keep solutions refrigerated until ready to use
  d. Allow a solution to hang for no more than 24 hours

    e. Monitor vital signs at least every 4 hours to detect any adverse reactions to infusion

    f. To help assess the effectiveness of TPN therapy, weigh the client daily while he's gaining weight (less frequently once his weight has stabilized)

    g. Test urine for glucose, ketones, and specific gravity every 4 to 6 hours to monitor for glucosuria and ketonuria

    h. Inspect the catheter insertion site every 8 hours if the client has a transparent dressing, or during dressing changes if the client has a gauze dressing; change dressings according to institutional policy

    i. Check infusion rate and administration system every hour, or according to institutional policy

    j. Change tubing and filters daily, or according to institutional policy

    k. Assist the client with walking if he's able, or with range-of-motion exercises if he's bedridden

    l. Maintain oral hygiene to prevent problems with the buccal cavity

    m. As ordered, discontinue TPN gradually—typically at a rate of 1,000 ml/day—while increasing oral or enteral feedings

    n. Confirm that an alternative feeding route is available before discontinuing TPN

    o. Do not force the client to eat during the weaning period; he probably will have little appetite

    p. Monitor the client's nutritional status during the weaning period by keeping an accurate record of food intake, including calorie count

    q. Maintain patency of the central catheter line if it has been left in place after discontinuing TPN

    r. Assist the physician in removing the central catheter line, as necessary

    s. After removal of the line, assess the catheterization site for proper wound healing

    t. If home TPN therapy is prescribed, instruct the client and his family on proper management techniques

6. Nursing implications for administering fat emulsions through TPN

    a. Inspect the bottle of fat emulsion for separation or an oily appearance; if present, do not administer

    b. Do not shake the bottle of fat emulsion or combine it with other solutions

    c. Hang the fat emulsion container higher than amino acid and dextrose solution containers, because fat emulsion has a higher specific gravity

    d. Do not use an in-line filter when administering fat emulsions; the fat particles will not pass through the 0.22 mcg cellulose filter usually used in TPN

    e. Use only the tubing supplied with the fat emulsion, to prevent possible interaction with plasticizers

   f. Begin by administering a test dose of 1 ml/min for 15 to 30 minutes, and observe the client's tolerance. If no reaction occurs, increase the infusion slowly until the desired flow rate is achieved

   g. Observe for immediate adverse reactions to fat emulsions, such as fever, flushing and sweating, insomnia, dizziness, nausea, vomiting, headache, chest and back pains, dyspnea, and cyanosis; these effects may occur within 2½ hours after initiating the infusion

   h. Observe for delayed adverse reactions, such as hepatomegaly, splenomegaly, thrombocytopenia, hyperlipidemia, seizures, shock, jaundice, and leukopenia

   i. Notify the physician immediately of any adverse reaction

   j. Be aware that fat emulsion should be used within 12 hours after starting the infusion; do not allow fat emulsion to hang for longer than 12 hours to prevent possible contamination

## Points to Remember

Parenteral nutrition is delivered intravenously through a peripheral or central vein.

Parenteral nutrition provides adequate nutritional intake when enteral nutrition is insufficient or contraindicated.

Parenteral nutrition can supply all the basic required nutrients: protein, carbohydrates, lipids, vitamins, and minerals.

The specific composition of parenteral solutions depends on the client's nutritional requirements and health status.

Peripheral parenteral nutrition (PPN) is considered a safer method of supplying nutrients than total parenteral nutrition (TPN) through a central vein; however, PPN usually is contraindicated for nutritionally depleted clients or clients with greatly increased nutritional requirements because of hypermetabolic states.

TPN, the most complex and expensive method available for providing nutrients, can be used to meet nutritional requirements for a prolonged period.

## Glossary

**Hepatomegaly**—enlargement of the liver

**Hyperalimentation**—intravenous feeding that supplies nutrients in excess of maintenance needs

**Hyperosmolar solution**—solution having an osmotic concentration above that of blood

**Isotonic solution**—solution having the same concentration of particles as another solution; exerts the same osmotic pressure, causing no net flow of water across the cell membrane

**Splenomegaly**—enlargement of the spleen

**Thrombocytopenia**—abnormal decrease in the number of circulating platelets

# Malnutrition

## Learning Objectives

After studying this section, the reader should be able to:

● Describe the general characteristics of malnutrition.

● Describe the general characteristics of obesity.

● Discuss important nursing implications related to obesity.

● Compare and contrast the three basic types of protein-energy malnutrition (PEM): iatrogenic PEM, kwashiorkor, and marasmus.

● Discuss important nursing implications related to all forms of PEM.

## XXVI. Malnutrition

### A. Introduction
1. *Malnutrition* is a general term literally meaning "bad" nutrition
2. *Malnutrition* refers to a deficit, excess, or imbalance of one or more essential nutrients
3. Conditions related to malnutrition include:
   a. Overnutrition: consumption of excessive food or nutrients, as occurs in obesity, megadoses of vitamins leading to toxicity, and overhydration
   b. Undernutrition: inadequate ingestion of nutrients, as in conditions such as protein-energy malnutrition (PEM), vitamin deficiencies, and dehydration
4. Mild malnutrition can interfere somewhat with body processes, quality of life, and sense of well-being
5. Severe malnutrition can produce specific nutritional disorders that may lead to irreversible damage to the body and possibly even to death
6. Most often in the United States, nutritional deficiencies tend to be asymptomatic, because clinical signs of poor nutrition may not be observable unless the problem is long-standing and severe
7. Clients who are under stress from surgery, burns, trauma, or illness and who also are malnourished may lack the nutritional reserves to handle the stress of the illness or injury
8. Conditions associated with high metabolic needs, such as burns, are more frequently associated with undernutrition
9. Malnutrition may be caused by *endogenous* factors, such as faulty metabolism, or *exogenous* factors, such as inadequate dietary intake
10. Malnutrition may be classified as *primary,* resulting directly from inadequate or excessive dietary intake of one or more essential nutrients, or *secondary* (also referred to as conditioned malnutrition), resulting from altered body functions, such as malabsorption syndrome
11. Risk factors associated with malnutrition include:
    a. Low education level
    b. Poverty
    c. Mental or physical disabilities
    d. Old age
    e. Alcoholism
    f. Drug addiction
    g. Food faddism
    h. Institutionalization in acute-care or long-term health care facilities or in prisons

### B. Obesity
1. Introduction
   a. Obesity is defined as weight exceeding 20% of the ideal body weight (IBW) for height and body frame. Degrees range from mild obesity (20% to 40% over IBW) to morbid obesity (100% or more over IBW)

    b.  Obesity is one of the most serious nutritional problems affecting Americans. Approximately 88 million Americans are overweight, with 40 million of them considered clinically obese

    c.  Obesity cuts across all socioeconomic levels; it may affect anyone at any time during the life-cycle

    d.  Obesity is the most common nutritional disturbance of childhood. By conservative estimates, 10% to 12% of all prepubertal children in the United States are obese. Approximately 80% of obese children become obese adults

    e.  Although many studies have been done on causes and effective treatments, obesity remains poorly understood and resistant to treatment. Genetic, physiologic, psychological, and environmental factors all appear to play some role

    f.  Obesity decreases life expectancy and may negatively affect the quality of life

    g.  Major physiologic complications of obesity include cardiovascular disease; respiratory disorders; diabetes mellitus; fatty liver infiltration; gallstone formation; pain and discomfort in weight-bearing joints of the hips, knees, and lower spine; menstrual irregularities, infertility, and endometrial cancer; complications during pregnancy, labor, and delivery; and increased surgical risk

    h.  Possible psychosocial disadvantages of obesity include feelings of poor self-esteem; feelings of failure, depression, frustration, and rejection; and possible discrimination by others in social, educational, and employment settings

    i.  Relevant benefits of weight reduction may include decreased high blood pressure, improved cardiac function, improved pulmonary ventilation, reduced osteoarthritis and low-back pain, improved peripheral vascular circulation, lessened fatigue and an increase in energy, improved self-esteem and body image, and increased sociability and improved relationships, including sexual relationships

    j.  Available treatments for obesity include weight-reduction diets, behavior modification, cognitive restructuring, physical exercise, relaxation techniques, support groups, and surgical interventions, such as gastric bypass

2.  Etiology: Excessive caloric-intake to energy-expenditure ratio

3.  Subjective assessment findings
    a.  Reported dysfunctional eating patterns
    b.  Stated sedentary activity level

4.  Objective assessment findings
    a.  Weight 20% or more over IBW for height and body frame
    b.  Triceps skinfold measurement greater than 15 mm in men and 25 mm in women
    c.  Observed dysfunctional eating patterns and sedentary activity level
    d.  Elevated serum cholesterol and serum triglyceride levels

5. Nursing implications
   a. Assess for causative and contributing factors that lead to weight gain
   b. Ascertain how the client perceives himself, food, and the act of eating
   c. Discuss with the client his motivation for wanting to lose weight
   d. Calculate the client's total caloric intake and energy expenditure
   e. Instruct the client to keep a food diary that includes all foods and fluids ingested daily and specifies amounts, times, places, companions, and feelings associated with eating
   f. Based on this diary, review the client's eating behaviors and identify necessary modifications
   g. Assess the client's knowledge of dietary needs and nutritional principles
   h. Review the client's daily activity and exercise program and suggest modifications, as necessary
   i. Working within accepted nutritional guidelines (and the client's physician's guidelines, if applicable), help the client determine the best weight-reduction diet for him
   j. Work with the client to set realistic goals for weekly weight loss
   k. Review the importance of a nutritionally balanced diet
   l. Stress the need for adequate fluid intake during weight loss to maintain renal function and promote excretion of wastes
   m. Help the client choose tasty, nutritious foods that are within his financial budget
   n. Encourage the client to include a variety of foods in his diet to decrease boredom and improve the chance of success
   o. Realistically point out the difficulties of weight loss and provide positive reinforcement
   p. Discuss ways of dealing with emotional stress that don't involve eating
   q. Involve the client and his family in the treatment plan as much as possible
   r. Refer the client to support groups or group therapy, as appropriate

C. **Protein energy malnutrition (PEM): General information**
   1. PEM is a type of primary malnutrition, also known as protein-calorie malnutrition
   2. PEM describes a spectrum of disorders resulting from either prolonged or chronic inadequate protein or caloric intake or from high metabolic protein and energy requirements
   3. With inadequate protein or caloric intake, the body meets its energy needs by breaking down and using stored proteins and fats
   4. Disorders commonly associated with PEM include cancer, GI disorders, chronic heart failure, alcoholism, and conditions with high metabolic needs, such as burns and infections
   5. Serious implications of PEM include:
      a. Reduced synthesis of enzymes and plasma proteins
      b. Increased susceptibility to infection

    c. Physical and mental growth deficiency in children
    d. Severe diarrhea and malabsorption
    e. Numerous secondary nutritional deficiencies
    f. Delayed wound healing
    g. Mental lassitude

6. PEM contributes to morbidity and mortality rates
7. Treatment measures for clients with PEM typically inlcude:
    a. Initiating a diet high in calories and protein and supplemented with enteral feedings
    b. Correcting fluid and electrolyte imbalances
    c. Treating any infection secondary to compromised immune function
    d. Initiating total parenteral nutrition (TPN) in severe PEM
8. PEM occurs in three basic forms:
    a. Iatrogenic PEM
    b. Kwashiorkor
    c. Marasmus
9. Nursing implications for all forms of PEM
    a. Assess baseline nutritional status, including dietary history and any complaints of recent weight loss
    b. Assess for causative and contributing factors, such as difficulty chewing or swallowing; and physical barriers, such as poverty, isolation, lack of transportation, ill-fitting dentures, or mental instability
    c. Observe client for any food intolerances or aversions
    d. Assess for possible drug interactions, allergies, and overuse of laxatives or diuretics that may alter nutritional status
    e. Assess for any psychological, social, and cultural factors that may influence nutritional status and help identify clients at risk
    f. Take baseline anthropometric measurements and monitor periodically to help evaluate the effectiveness of therapy
    g. Review laboratory test findings, specifically serum transferrin and albumin levels and total lymphocyte count (TLC)
    h. Provide appropriate treatment to help correct or control underlying causative factors such as cancer or anorexia
    i. Note total daily caloric intake, and calculate basal energy expenditure; monitor calorie count and weight daily
    j. Provide dietary modifications, as indicated and as tolerated by the client, such as increasing intake of protein, calories, and fats
    k. Provide small feedings of foods the client can easily chew, swallow, and digest
    l. Encourage the client and his family to choose foods with high nutritional value
    m. Provide a pleasant, relaxing environment for meals
    n. Provide for hygiene, such as hand-washing and oral hygiene, before and after meals

o. Promote adequate fluid intake; may limit fluids 1 hour before meals to decrease feelings of fullness and enhance appetite
p. Provide nutritional supplements as ordered
q. As ordered, administer agents that help alleviate conditions that interfere with nutritional status, such as antacids, anticholinergics, antiemetics, and antidiarrheals
r. Work with the client to develop a realistic goal for weight gain
s. Help the client develop a regular exercise and stress-reduction program, as appropriate
t. Consult with the dietitian or nutritional support team as necessary
u. Teach the client and his family the importance of well-balanced nutrition to avoid further problems with PEM
v. As needed, help the client and his family secure and use available resources, such as food stamps, to improve nutritional intake

**D. Iatrogenic PEM: Specific information**
1. Introduction
   a. Iatrogenic PEM most commonly occurs in clients hospitalized longer than 2 weeks, and may affect more than 15% of clients hospitalized in acute care centers
   b. Studies show that a client's nutritional status often deteriorates during hospitalization, which can lead to iatrogenic PEM
   c. In hospitalized clients, iatrogenic PEM can result from acts and omissions by health care providers and from institutional policies and practices that undermine optimal nutritional care
   d. Nurses involved in routine client care are those most likely to observe the early signs and symptoms of PEM
2. Etiology
   a. Exogenous causes, such as prolonged or chronically inadequate intake of protein, calories, or both
   b. Endogenous causes, such as excessively increased protein and caloric requirements from hypermetabolic or malabsorption states
3. Subjective assessment findings
   a. Reported inadequate food intake (less than recommended dietary allowances [RDAs]) with or without weight loss
   b. Stated lack of interest in or aversion to eating
   c. Reported altered taste sensation
   d. Complaints of abdominal discomfort or cramping (with or without underlying pathologic conditions)
   e. Perceived inability to eat
   f. Reported lack of information, misinformation, or misconceptions about nutrition
4. Objective assessment findings
   a. Body weight 10% to 20% or more below IBW for height and frame size
   b. Loss of weight with adequate food intake

      c. Poor muscle tone
      d. Weakness of muscles required for chewing or swallowing
      e. Sore, inflamed buccal cavity
      f. Capillary fragility
      g. Hyperactive bowel sounds
      h. Diarrhea or steatorrhea
      i. Pale conjunctivae and mucous membranes
      j. Decreased subcutaneous fat and muscle mass with triceps skinfold (TSF) measurement and mid-arm circumference (MAC) less than 60% of standard
      k. Amenorrhea
      l. Tachycardia on minimal exercise and bradycardia at rest
      m. Mental irritability or confusion
      n. Decreased serum albumin level
      o. Decreased serum transferrin level or total iron-binding capacity (TIBC)
      p. Decreased TLC

5. Nursing implications for iatrogenic PEM
      a. Keep in mind that clients who are hospitalized for longer than 2 weeks or are debilitated are at a high risk for developing iatrogenic PEM
      b. Monitor laboratory test findings and fluid and electrolyte balance closely for improvement
      c. Assist the client with menu selection, offering guidance as necessary for nutritious foods
      d. Examine the client's tray to determine intake; record client's intake and ability to tolerate the meal
      e. Offer assistance with feeding, as necessary
      f. Anticipate the need for possible feeding alternatives, such as enteral or parenteral nutrition; explain the rationale to the client
      g. Teach the client about PEM and measures to control and prevent it
      h. Encourage the client and family to adhere to a plan for medical follow-up
      i. See "Nursing implications for all forms of PEM," page 188

## E. Kwashiorkor: Specific information

1. Introduction
      a. Kwashiorkor (literally "the disease of the deposed baby when the next one is born") is a form of PEM caused by severe protein deficiency
      b. It most commonly affects children age 1 to 3 years as they are weaned from the breast when another child is born
      c. Kwashiorkor most commonly occurs in areas where economic, social, and cultural factors combine to prevent adequate protein intake, such as in most of the Middle and Far Eastern countries, India, all the countries and territories of Africa south of the Sahara, and 19 of the 21 countries in the Americas

    d. In the United States, it most commonly occurs secondary to malabsorption disorders, cancer and cancer therapies, kidney disease, hypermetabolic illness, and iatrogenic causes

    e. It is associated with a high mortality rate, with death typically occurring before age 5

2. Etiology

    a. Kwashiorkor is hypothesized to occur when the body cannot adapt to decreased protein intake because of superimposed illness or infection

    b. It is caused by inadequate intake of good-quality protein when caloric intake is marginally adequate

3. Subjective assessment findings

    a. Reported inadequate dietary intake of protein foods

    b. Stated recent weaning of child from the breast

    c. Reported poor appetite

4. Objective assessment findings

    a. Generalized illness, usually with fever

    b. Retarded growth and malnutrition

    c. Weight loss and muscle wasting; may be masked by a well-nourished appearance or edema in the face and lower body; "pot-bellied" appearance

    d. Sparse, thin, soft hair, possibly with parallel grey, red, or blond streaks (flag sign)

    e. Mucous membrane changes, such as cracks in the corners of the mouth, ulcerations, tongue atrophy

    f. Depigmentation of hair and skin

    g. Apathy, irritability

    h. Decreased serum albumin levels

    i. Decreased TIBC, serum transferrin levels, and TLC

5. Nursing implications for Kwashiorkor

    a. Identify children at risk for kwashiorkor

    b. Question the mother or primary caregiver about the child's dietary intake

    c. Assess for objective signs of kwashiorkor

    d. Perform anthropometric measurements; use as a baseline and to evaluate therapy

    e. Review diagnostic findings; monitor diagnostic tests frequently for changes and improvements

    f. Provide assistance in correcting underlying causes of nonavailability of good protein

    g. Consult with dietitian or nutritional support team as necessary to assist the mother or primary caregiver with supplying adequate diet

    h. Instruct the mother or primary caregiver in foods with high nutritional value

    i. Refer the client and family to social services, if necessary, for financial assistance with food purchases

    j. See "Nursing implications for all forms of PEM," page 190

F. **Marasmus: Specific information**
1. Introduction
   a. *Marasmus,* also known as general malnutrition or energy-deficient malnutrition, is a form of PEM most commonly affecting infants ages 6 to 18 months
   b. Its incidence is widespread and not confined to underprivileged countries
   c. The infant's parents typically are indigent, uneducated, or mentally or emotionally disturbed
   d. Marasmus may also strike elderly poor people or young adults who have dieted excessively
2. Etiology
   a. Marasmus is hypothesized to be a normal adaptive response to starvation
   b. It is caused by chronic lack of calories, proteins, and nearly all other nutrients
3. Subjective assessment findings
   a. Reported chronic, inadequate food intake
   b. Reported chronic loss of appetite
4. Objective assessment findings
   a. Emaciated appearance with little or no edema
   b. Muscle wasting with loss of subcutaneous fat
   c. Subnormal body temperature
   d. Failure to thrive
   e. TSF less than 3 mm
   f. Mid-arm muscle circumference (MAMC) less than 15 cm
   g. Normal serum albumin and transferrin levels
5. Nursing implications
   a. Identify children at risk for marasmus
   b. Assess diet for good-quality protein and caloric intake; question the mother or primary caregiver about the child's diet
   c. Evaluate the child for possible underlying causes of marasmus, such as malabsorption
   d. Instruct the mother or primary caregiver in high-nutrition foods
   e. Refer the client and family to community and social service agencies for needed financial assistance and follow-up
   f. See "Nursing implications for all forms of PEM," page 190

## Points to Remember

Malnutrition refers to a deficit, excess, or imbalance of one or more essential nutrients.

Mild malnutrition can interfere somewhat with body processes, quality of life, and sense of well-being. Severe malnutrition can produce specific nutritional disorders that may lead to irreversible damage to the body and possibly even to death.

Obesity is one of the most serious nutritional problems affecting Americans.

The nurse is usually in the best position to recognize clients at high risk for nutritional disorders and to provide the necessary nutritional care to help prevent serious effects of malnutrition.

The nurse's effectiveness in caring for clients with PEM or obesity depends on a knowledge of nutritional principles, awareness of factors that have nutritional implications, and ability to communicate observations to others on the health care team.

## Glossary

**Kwashiorkor**—form of protein-energy malnutrition (PEM) produced by severe protein deficiency

**Malnutrition**—deficit, excess, or imbalance of one or more essential nutrients

**Marasmus**—one form of PEM most commonly affecting infants ages 6 to 18 months

**Obesity**—weight exceeding 20% of the IBW for height and body frame

**Protein-energy malnutrition (PEM)**—malnutrition resulting from insufficient intake or use of protein, calories, or both

# Appendices

## Appendix A

### RECOMMENDED DIETARY ALLOWANCES[a]

| AGE | INFANTS (both sexes) | | CHILDREN (both sexes) | | | MALES | | |
|---|---|---|---|---|---|---|---|---|
| | 0-6 mo | 6-12 mo | 1-3 yr | 4-6 yr | 7-10 yr | 11-14 yr | 15-18 yr | 19-22 yr |
| Energy (kcal) | kg × 115 | kg × 105 | 1,300 | 1,700 | 2,400 | 2,700 | 2,800 | 2,900 |
| Protein (g) | kg × 2.2 | kg × 2.0 | 23 | 30 | 34 | 45 | 56 | 56 |
| **Fat-soluble vitamins** | | | | | | | | |
| Vit. A (mg re)[b] | 420 | 400 | 400 | 500 | 700 | 1,000 | 1,000 | 1,000 |
| Vit. D (mcg)[c] | 10 | 10 | 10 | 10 | 10 | 10 | 10 | 7.5 |
| Vit. E (mg $\alpha$te)[d] | 3 | 4 | 5 | 6 | 7 | 8 | 10 | 10 |
| **Water-soluble vitamins** | | | | | | | | |
| Vitamin C (mg) | 35 | 35 | 45 | 45 | 45 | 50 | 60 | 60 |
| Folacin (mcg)[e] | 30 | 45 | 100 | 200 | 300 | 400 | 400 | 400 |
| Niacin (mg NE)[f] | 6 | 8 | 9 | 11 | 16 | 18 | 18 | 19 |
| Riboflavin (mg) | 0.4 | 0.6 | 0.8 | 1.0 | 1.4 | 1.6 | 1.7 | 1.7 |
| Thiamin (mg) | 0.3 | 0.5 | 0.7 | 0.9 | 1.2 | 1.4 | 1.4 | 1.5 |
| Vitamin $B_6$ (mg) | 0.3 | 0.6 | 0.9 | 1.3 | 1.6 | 1.8 | 2.0 | 2.2 |
| Vitamin $B_{12}$ (mcg) | 0.5[g] | 1.5 | 2.0 | 2.5 | 3.0 | 3.0 | 3.0 | 3.0 |
| **Minerals** | | | | | | | | |
| Calcium (mg) | 360 | 540 | 800 | 800 | 800 | 1,200 | 1,200 | 800 |
| Phosphorus (mg) | 240 | 360 | 800 | 800 | 800 | 1,200 | 1,200 | 800 |
| Iodine (mcg) | 40 | 50 | 70 | 90 | 120 | 150 | 150 | 150 |
| Iron (mg) | 10 | 15 | 15 | 10 | 10 | 18 | 18 | 10 |
| Magnesium (mg) | 50 | 70 | 150 | 200 | 250 | 350 | 400 | 350 |
| Zinc (mg) | 3 | 5 | 10 | 10 | 10 | 15 | 15 | 15 |

[a]The allowances are intended to provide for individual variations among most normal persons as they live in the United States under usual environmental stresses. Diets should be based on a variety of common foods in order to provide other nutrients for which human requirements have been well defined.
[b]Retinol equivalents. 1 Retinol equivalent = 1 mcg retinol or 6 mcg beta carotene.
[c]As cholecalciferol. 10 mcg cholecalciferol = 400 IU vitamin D.
[d]Alpha tocopherol equivalents (Alpha TE). 1 mg d-Alpha-tocopherol = 1 Alpha TE.
[e]The folacin allowances refer to dietary sources as determined by *Lactobacillus casei* assay after treatment with enzymes ("conjugases") to make polyglutamyl forms of the vitamin available to the test organism.
[f]1 NE (niacin equivalent) is equal to 1 mg of niacin or 60 mg of dietary tryptophan.
[g]The RDA for vitamin $B_{12}$ in infants is based on average concentration of the vitamin in human milk. The allowances after weaning are based on energy intake (as recommended by the American Academy of Pediatrics) and consideration of other factors such as intestinal absorption.

| 23-50 yr | 51+ yr | FEMALES | | | | | Pregnant | Lactating |
|---|---|---|---|---|---|---|---|---|
| | | 11-14 yr | 15-18 yr | 19-22 yr | 23-50 yr | 51+ yr | | |
| 2,700 | 2,400[i] | 2,200 | 2,100 | 2,100 | 2,000 | 1,800[i] | +300 | +500 |
| 56 | 56 | 46 | 46 | 44 | 44 | 44 | +30 | +20 |
| 1,000 | 1,000 | 800 | 800 | 800 | 800 | 800 | +200 | +400 |
| 5.0 | 5.0 | 10 | 10 | 7.5 | 5.0 | 5.0 | +5.0 | +5.0 |
| 10 | 10 | 8 | 8 | 8 | 8 | 8 | +2 | +3 |
| 60 | 60 | 50 | 60 | 60 | 60 | 60 | +20 | +40 |
| 400 | 400 | 400 | 400 | 400 | 400 | 400 | +400 | +100 |
| 18 | 16 | 15 | 14 | 14 | 13 | 13 | +2 | +5 |
| 1.6 | 1.4 | 1.3 | 1.3 | 1.3 | 1.2 | 1.2 | +0.3 | +0.5 |
| 1.4 | 1.2 | 1.1 | 1.1 | 1.1 | 1.0 | 1.0 | +0.4 | +0.5 |
| 2.2 | 2.2 | 1.8 | 2.0 | 2.0 | 2.0 | 2.0 | +0.6 | +0.5 |
| 3.0 | 3.0 | 3.0 | 3.0 | 3.0 | 3.0 | 3.0 | +1.0 | +1.0 |
| 800 | 800 | 1,200 | 1,200 | 800 | 800 | 800 | +400 | +400 |
| 800 | 800 | 1,200 | 1,200 | 800 | 800 | 800 | +400 | +400 |
| 150 | 150 | 150 | 150 | 150 | 150 | 150 | +25 | +50 |
| 10 | 10 | 18 | 18 | 18 | 18 | 10 | h | h |
| 350 | 350 | 300 | 300 | 300 | 300 | 300 | +150 | +150 |
| 15 | 15 | 15 | 15 | 15 | 15 | 15 | +5 | +10 |

hThe increased requirements during pregnancy cannot be met by the iron content of habitual American diets nor by the existing iron stores of many women; therefore, the use of 30 to 60 mg of supplemental iron is recommended. Iron needs during lactation are not substantially different from those of nonpregnant women, but continued supplementation of the mother for 2 to 3 months after parturition is advisable in order to replenish stores depleted by pregnancy.
iThis is the recommended energy intake for individuals aged 51 to 75. While nutrient needs for older individuals have not been established, the U.S. RDA energy intake for men over age 75 is 2,050 Kcal, and for women, 1,600 Kcal.

# Appendix B

## RECOMMENDED NUTRIENT INTAKE FOR CANADIANS[a,b]

| | INFANTS (both sexes) | | | | CHILDREN (both sexes) | | | MALES | | | | |
|---|---|---|---|---|---|---|---|---|---|---|---|---|
| **AGE** | 0-2 months | 3-5 | 6-8 | 9-11 | 1 years | 2-3 | 4-6 | 7-9 years | 10-12 | 13-15 | 16-18 | 19-24 |
| Protein (g/day)[c] | 11[h] | 14[h] | 17[h] | 18 | 19 | 22 | 26 | 30 | 38 | 50 | 55 | 58 |
| **Fat-soluble vitamins** | | | | | | | | | | | | |
| Vitamin A (RE/day)[d] | 400 | 400 | 400 | 400 | 400 | 400 | 500 | 700 | 800 | 900 | 1,000 | 1,000 |
| Vitamin D (mcg/day)[e] | 10 | 10 | 10 | 10 | 10 | 5 | 5 | 2.5 | 2.5 | 2.5 | 2.5 | 2.5 |
| Vitamin E (mg/day)[f] | 3 | 3 | 3 | 3 | 3 | 4 | 5 | 7 | 8 | 9 | 10 | 10 |
| **Water-soluble vitamins** | | | | | | | | | | | | |
| Vitamin C (mg/day) | 20 | 20 | 20 | 20 | 20 | 20 | 25 | 35 | 40 | 50 | 55 | 60 |
| Folacin (mcg/day)[g] | 50 | 50 | 50 | 55 | 65 | 80 | 90 | 125 | 170 | 150 | 185 | 210 |
| Vitamin $B_{12}$ (mcg/day) | 0.3 | 0.3 | 0.3 | 0.3 | 0.3 | 0.4 | 0.5 | 0.8 | 1.0 | 1.5 | 1.9 | 2.0 |
| **Minerals** | | | | | | | | | | | | |
| Calcium (mg/day) | 350 | 350 | 400 | 400 | 500 | 500 | 600 | 700 | 900 | 1,100 | 900 | 800 |
| Magnesium (mg/day) | 30 | 40 | 50 | 50 | 55 | 70 | 90 | 110 | 150 | 210 | 250 | 240 |
| Iron (mg/day) | 0.4[i] | 5 | 7 | 7 | 6 | 6 | 6 | 7 | 10 | 12 | 10 | 8 |
| Iodine (mcg/day) | 25 | 35 | 40 | 45 | 55 | 65 | 85 | 110 | 125 | 160 | 160 | 160 |
| Zinc (mg/day) | 2[j] | 3 | 3 | 3 | 4 | 4 | 5 | 6 | 7 | 9 | 9 | 9 |

[a]Recommended intakes of energy and of certain nutrients are not listed in this table because of the nature of the variables upon which they are based. The figures for energy are estimates of average requirements for expected patterns of activity. For nutrients not shown, the following amounts are recommended: thaimin, 0.4 mg/1000 kcal (0.48 mg/5000 kJ); riboflavin, 0.5 mg/1000 kcal (0.6 mg/5000 kJ); niacin, 7.2 NE/1000 kcal (8.6 NE/5000 kJ); vitamin B6, 15 µg, as pyridoxine, per gram of protein; phosphorus, same as calcium.
[b]Recommended intakes during periods of growth are taken as appropriate for individuals representative of the mid-point in each age group. All recommended intakes are designed to cover individual variations in essentially all of a healthy population subsisting upon a variety of common foods available in Canada.
[c]The primary units are grams per kilogram of body weight. The figures shown here are only examples.
[d]One retinol equivalent (RE) corresponds to the biological activity of 1 µg of retinol, 6 µg of β-carotene or 12 µg of other carotenes.
[e]Expressed as cholecalciferol or ergocalciferol.
[f]Expressed as $d$-α-tocopherol equivalents, relative to which β- and γ-tocopherol and α-tocotrienol have activities of 0.5, 0.1 and 0.3 respectively.

| | | FEMALES | | | | | | | | Pregnant (additional) | | | Lactating (additional) |
|---|---|---|---|---|---|---|---|---|---|---|---|---|---|
| 50-74 | 75+ | 7-9 years | 10-12 | 13-15 | 16-18 | 19-24 | 25-49 | 50-74 | 75+ | 1st trimester | 2nd | 3rd | |
| 60 | 57 | 30 | 40 | 42 | 43 | 43 | 44 | 47 | 47 | 15 | 20 | 25 | 20 |
| 1,000 | 1,000 | 700 | 800 | 800 | 800 | 800 | 800 | 800 | 800 | 100 | 100 | 100 | 400 |
| 2.5 | 2.5 | 2.5 | 2.5 | 2.5 | 2.5 | 2.5 | 2.5 | 2.5 | 2.5 | 2.5 | 2.5 | 2.5 | 2.5 |
| 7 | 6 | 6 | 7 | 7 | 7 | 7 | 6 | 6 | 5 | 2 | 2 | 2 | 3 |
| 60 | 60 | 30 | 40 | 45 | 45 | 45 | 45 | 45 | 45 | 0 | 20 | 20 | 30 |
| 220 | 205 | 125 | 180 | 145 | 160 | 175 | 175 | 190 | 190 | 305 | 305 | 305 | 120 |
| 2.0 | 2.0 | 0.8 | 1.0 | 1.5 | 1.9 | 2.0 | 2.0 | 2.0 | 2.0 | 1.0 | 1.0 | 1.0 | 0.5 |
| 800 | 800 | 700 | 1,000 | 800 | 700 | 700 | 700 | 800 | 800 | 500 | 500 | 500 | 500 |
| 250 | 230 | 110 | 160 | 200 | 215 | 200 | 200 | 210 | 220 | 15 | 20 | 25 | 80 |
| 8 | 8 | 7 | 10 | 13 | 14 | 14 | 14[k] | 7 | 7 | 6 | 6 | 6 | 0 |
| 160 | 160 | 95 | 110 | 160 | 160 | 160 | 160 | 160 | 160 | 25 | 25 | 25 | 50 |
| 9 | 9 | 6 | 7 | 8 | 8 | 8 | 8 | 8 | 8 | 0 | 1 | 2 | 6 |

[g]Assumption that the protein is from breast milk or is of the same biological value as that of breast milk and that between 3 and 9 months adjustment for the quality of the protein is made.
[i]Based on the assumption that breast milk is the source of iron for the first 2 months.
[j]Based on the assumption that breast milk is the source of zinc for the first 2 months.
[k]After menopause the recommended intake is 7 mg/day.

## Appendix C

## U.S. RECOMMENDED DAILY ALLOWANCES (U.S. RDAs)

| NUTRIENT | ADULTS AND CHILDREN AGE 4 OR OLDER | CHILDREN UNDER AGE 4 | INFANTS UNDER AGE 1 | PREGNANT OR LACTATING WOMEN |
|---|---|---|---|---|
| *Vitamin A | 5,000 I.U. | 2,500 | 1,500 | 8,000 |
| Vitamin D | 400** I.U. | 400 | 400 | 400 |
| Vitamin E | 30 I.U. | 10 | 5 | 30 |
| *Vitamin C | 60 mg | 40 | 35 | 60 |
| Folic acid | 0.4 mg | 0.2 | 0.1 | 0.8 |
| *Thiamine | 1.5 mg | 0.7 | 0.5 | 1.7 |
| *Riboflavin | 1.7 mg | 0.8 | 0.6 | 2.0 |
| *Niacin | 20 mg | 9.0 | 8.0 | 20 |
| Vitamin $B_6$ | 2.0 mg | 0.7 | 0.4 | 2.5 |
| Vitamin $B_{12}$ | 6.0 mcg | 3.0 | 2.0 | 8.0 |
| Biotin | 0.3 mg | 0.15 | 0.5 | 0.3 |
| Pantothenic acid | 10 mg | 5.0 | 3.0 | 10 |
| *Calcium | 1.0 g | 0.8 | 0.6 | 1.3 |
| Phosphorous | 1.0 g | 0.8 | 0.5 | 1.3 |
| Iodine | 150 mcg | 70 | 45 | 150 |
| *Iron | 18 mg | 10 | 15 | 18 |
| Magnesium | 400 mg | 200 | 70 | 450 |
| Copper | 2.0 mg | 1.0 | 0.6 | 2.0 |
| Zinc | 15 mg | 8.0 | 5.0 | 15 |
| + Protein | 45 g | 20 | 18 | 65-75 |

* Manufacturer must list these nutrients on nutrition labels.
** Vitamin D is optional in supplements for adults and children age 4 or older.
+ If protein quality is equal to or greater than high-quality milk protein.

From *Vitamins and Minerals*. American Family Health Institute publication. Springhouse, Pa.: Springhouse Corp., 1986, p. 25.

# Appendix D

## HEIGHT AND WEIGHT TABLES

Weights are for adults ages 25 to 59 and are based on lowest mortality. Weight in pounds is according to frame size, including indoor clothing (5 pounds for men and 3 pounds for women); height assumes shoes with 1" heels.

### MEN

| Height | Weight | | |
| --- | --- | --- | --- |
| | Small frame | Medium frame | Large frame |
| 5'2" | 128-134 | 131-141 | 138-150 |
| 5'3" | 130-136 | 133-143 | 140-153 |
| 5'4" | 132-138 | 135-145 | 142-156 |
| 5'5" | 134-140 | 137-148 | 144-160 |
| 5'6" | 136-142 | 139-151 | 146-164 |
| 5'7" | 138-145 | 142-154 | 149-168 |
| 5'8" | 140-148 | 145-157 | 152-172 |
| 5'9" | 142-151 | 148-160 | 155-176 |
| 5'10" | 144-154 | 151-163 | 158-180 |
| 5'11" | 146-157 | 154-166 | 161-184 |
| 6'0" | 149-160 | 157-170 | 164-188 |
| 6'1" | 152-164 | 160-174 | 168-192 |
| 6'2" | 155-168 | 164-178 | 172-197 |
| 6'3" | 158-172 | 167-182 | 176-202 |
| 6'4" | 162-176 | 171-187 | 181-207 |

### WOMEN

| Height | Weight | | |
| --- | --- | --- | --- |
| | Small frame | Medium frame | Large frame |
| 4'10" | 102-111 | 109-121 | 118-131 |
| 4'11" | 103-113 | 111-123 | 120-134 |
| 5'0" | 104-115 | 113-126 | 122-137 |
| 5'1" | 106-118 | 115-129 | 125-140 |
| 5'2" | 108-121 | 118-132 | 128-143 |
| 5'3" | 111-124 | 121-135 | 131-147 |
| 5'4" | 114-127 | 124-138 | 134-151 |
| 5'5" | 117-130 | 127-141 | 137-155 |
| 5'6" | 120-133 | 130-144 | 140-159 |
| 5'7" | 123-136 | 133-147 | 143-163 |
| 5'8" | 126-139 | 136-150 | 146-167 |
| 5'9" | 129-142 | 139-153 | 149-170 |
| 5'10" | 132-145 | 142-156 | 152-173 |
| 5'11" | 135-148 | 145-159 | 155-176 |
| 6'0" | 138-151 | 148-162 | 158-179 |

Courtesy of the Metropolitan Life Insurance Co., New York (based on 1983 study).

## Appendix E

### SELECTED DRUG EFFECTS ON NUTRIENTS

Food can influence drug actions in the body; conversely, drugs can affect specific nutrient absorption or excretion by the body. Some drugs enhance nutrient absorption, whereas others can produce nutrient toxicity or possible deficiency. Below is a listing of selected drugs and their effects on nutrients.

| DRUG | NUTRIENT | DRUG EFFECT |
|---|---|---|
| Aspirin | Folic acid | Interferes with absorption and use; promotes faster folate excretion |
| | Vitamin C | Increases urine excretion |
| | Vitamin K | Depletes body stores; increases urine excretion |
| Adrenocorticosteroids | Vitamin D | Decreases metabolism |
| | Zinc, vitamin C, potassium, magnesium | Increases urine excretion |
| | Calcium | Decreases absorption; increases urine excretion |
| | Phosphorus, vitamin A, vitamin $B_6$ | Decreases absorption |
| | Glucose, triglycerides, cholesterol | Increases blood levels |
| Antacids | Vitamin D, iron, thiamin | Interferes with absorption and use |
| | Phosphorus | Interferes with absorption and use; increases excretion |
| Anticonvulsants | Folic acid | Interferes with absorption and use |
| | Vitamins D, K | Interferes with metabolism |
| Chloramphenicol | Lactose | Interferes with absorption |
| | Protein, vitamin K | Interferes with synthesis |
| | Riboflavin, pyridoxine, vitamin $B_{12}$ | Increases requirements |
| Chlorothiazides | Calcium | Increases absorption |
| | Carbohydrate | Decreases tolerance |
| | Riboflavin, potassium, zinc, magnesium | Increases excretion |
| Chlorthalidone | Zinc | Increases excretion |
| Cholestyramine | Vitamins A, D, E, K, $B_{12}$, folic acid, iron | Interferes with absorption and use |
| | Calcium | Increases excretion |
| Colchicine | Vitamins A, $B_{12}$, fat, lactose | Interferes with absorption and use |
| | Sodium, potassium | Increases excretion |

## SELECTED DRUG EFFECTS ON NUTRIENTS continued

| DRUG | NUTRIENT | DRUG EFFECT |
|---|---|---|
| Digitalis | Glucose | Interferes with absorption and use |
| | Magnesium | Increases excretion |
| Ethacrynic acid | Potassium, sodium, magnesium, calcium | Increases excretion |
| Isoniazid | Vitamin $B_6$ | Decreases metabolism |
| | Iron | Increases absorption |
| Laxatives | Vitamins D, K, glucose, calcium | Interferes with absorption and use |
| | Potassium, sodium, calcium, magnesium, water-soluble vitamins | Increases excretion |
| Levodopa | Vitamin $B_{12}$ | Interferes with absorption and use |
| | Sodium, potassium | Increases excretion |
| MAO inhibitors | Tyramine, tyrosine | Blocks metabolism |
| Hydrochlorothiazide | Magnesium, potassium, zinc, riboflavin | Increases urine excretion |
| Methotrexate | Vitamin $B_{12}$ | Interferes with absorption |
| | Fat, carotene, lactose, cholesterol | Causes malabsorption |
| Mineral oil | Vitamins A, D, E, K, phosphorus, calcium | Interferes with absorption and use |
| Neomycin | Vitamins A, $B_{12}$, K, protein, lactose, fat, calcium, iron | Interferes with absorption and use |
| | Sodium, potassium | Increases excretion |
| Oral contraceptives | Folic acid, vitamin $B_6$ | Increases excretion |
| | Riboflavin, vitamin $B_{12}$ | Depletes body stores |
| | Vitamin C | Decreases absorption; increases metabolism |
| | Copper | Increases absorption |
| Penicillin G Potassium | Vitamin K | Decreases synthesis |
| | Potassium | Increases excretion |
| | Folic acid, vitamin $B_{12}$, calcium, magnesium, glucose, carotene, cholesterol | Decreases absorption |

continued

**SELECTED DRUG EFFECTS ON NUTRIENTS** continued

| DRUG | NUTRIENT | DRUG EFFECT |
|---|---|---|
| Phenobarbital | Vitamin D, thiamin, folic acid, calcium | Interferes with absorption and use |
|  | Vitamin C | Increases excretion |
| Phenytoin | Calcium | Interferes with absorption and use |
|  | Vitamins C, D | Increases excretion |
|  | Folic acid | Decreases mucosal uptake |
| Potassium chloride | Vitamin $B_{12}$ | Interferes with absorption |
| Primidone | Calcium, folic acid, vitamins $B_6$, $B_{12}$ | Decreases absorption |
| Sulfonamides | Folic acid, iron, vitamin $B_{12}$, calcium | Decreases absorption |
|  | Vitamin K | Reduces synthesis |
| Tetracyclines | Folic acid, calcium, vitamin $B_{12}$, magnesium, copper, iron, cobalt, manganese, zinc | Decreases absorption |
|  | Vitamin K | Decreases synthesis |
|  | Vitamin $B_6$ | Inactivates the vitamin |
| Thyroxine | Riboflavin | Interferes with absorption and use |
| Triamterene | Folic acid | Interferes with absorption and use |
|  | Calcium | Increases excretion |
| Warfarin | Vitamin K | Depresses synthesis |

## Appendix F

### SELECTED FOOD AND DRUG INTERACTIONS

Food and drug interactions can mean the difference between success or failure in drug therapy. Food can influence drug absorption and action in several ways, depending on the specific drugs and foods involved. Although food usually delays dissolution and absorption of orally administered drugs, most drugs are eventually absorbed and the patient receives the intended therapeutic effect. In some cases, however, food has an undesirable effect on therapy.

Food may also enhance drug absorption. By stimulating gastric acid secretion, for example, food in the stomach may enhance dissolution and absorption of acidic drugs.

The chart below lists the effect of food on specific drugs.

| FOOD EFFECT | DRUGS AFFECTED | |
|---|---|---|
| Delays absorption | • acetaminophen<br>• amoxicillin<br>• ampicillin<br>• belladonna compounds<br>• cephalexin<br>• digoxin | • monoamine oxidase inhibitors<br>• sulfisoxazole<br>• sulindac<br>• tetracyclines<br>• theophylline (with high-protein meals)<br>• tolmetin |
| Decreases absorption | • captopril<br>• lincomycin<br>• nafcillin sodium | • oxytetracycline<br>• rifampin |
| Delays or decreases absorption and reduces GI distress | • aspirin<br>• aminophylline<br>• fenoprofen calcium<br>• furosemide | • ibuprofen<br>• methotrexate<br>• phenobarbital |
| Increases absorption | • carbamazepine<br>• lithium<br>• propranolol | • theophylline (with high-carbohydrate meals) |
| Increases absorption and reduces GI distress | • hydrochlorothiazide<br>• nitrofurantoin | • phenytoin |
| Slows absorption; acid foods speed dissolution | • diazepam | |
| Decreases absorption | • erythromycin | |
| Delays absorption and minimizes vascular headaches | • isosorbide dinitrate | |

# Index

t refers to a table.

t refers to a table.

t refers to a table.